Life on Cripple Creek

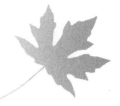

ESSAYS ON LIVING WITH
MULTIPLE SCLEROSIS

Dean Kramer

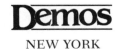

NEW YORK

Library of Congress Cataloging-in-Publication Data

Kramer, Dean, 1951-
  Life on Cripple Creek : essays on living with multiple sclerosis / Dean Kramer.
      p. ; cm.
    ISBN 1-888799-68-4 (pbk.)
    1. Kramer, Dean, 1951– Health. 2. Multiple sclerosis—Patients—United States—Biography.
    [DNLM: 1. Multiple Sclerosis—Personal Narratives. 2. Multiple Sclerosis—Popular Works. WL 360 K89L 2002]
  I. Title.
    RC377 .K735 2002
    362.1'96834'0093—dc21

                                        2002012435

Interior designed and typeset in Fairfield by Gopa & Ted2

Printed in Canada

Contents

Foreword
by Margot Russell

WHAT IS ORDINARY? How often we believe that we are living an ordinary day in an ordinary life; we are prone to viewing ourselves through the smallest lens of the telescope. But it's said that our lives are best defined by the myriad of details that mark our days: The first thing you thought when you awoke this morning, the song that you were humming as you made your way to work. Perhaps the largest part of who we are is revealed in this moment—in the way we are living right now.

The most endearing quality of the book you are holding, *Life on Cripple Creek*, is that Dean Kramer allows us to peek inside the windows of her rustic home in rural Pennsylvania and share a day in her life with a chronic illness. We follow her to the raspberry patch, we ride across the great expanse on her scooter, we laugh with her as she struggles to flee a swarm of bees. And what we come away with at the end of the day transforms us: Life's lessons are learned from the way we are being, and not necessarily from what we are doing. And when we keep our eyes wide open, what may seem ordinary can become our greatest gift.

Living life with multiple sclerosis is an incredible challenge. Our days are marked by unimaginable changes, and it's easy to focus on those things we've lost along the way. We wonder—in the light of our illness—who we are now and where the road may lead. Lost in these larger questions, we sometimes forget the beauty of the smallest gesture, the importance of seeing ourselves in the context of now, the certainty that the most profound lessons lie in the simplest of truths. What Dean shows us, then, as we wander up the hill, is that illness can transform us if we listen close enough. When we start to pay attention to our lives, when we cock our ears to the errant whispers in the wind, we begin to view ourselves in a different light. The nuances of illness—both subtle and provocative-become powerful tools in understanding and grappling with our inner selves.

"Illness as a gift" is a difficult metaphor to ascribe to, but it's often used to illustrate the wisdom gained from those who've walked that road. Often, those who journey with illness stumble upon life's larger truths and then find they are unwilling to trade the lessons learned along the way. *Life on Cripple Creek* brings you on that journey, leaving you back on your own doorstep; less afraid of the unknown, more certain that the true joys in life begin somewhere in your own backyard. The challenge lies in the excavation, the digging deep for the gifts of everyday.

Illness often becomes a filter, one that all life experience must pass through before it rearranges itself and settles into our consciousness. It is important, then, to separate our true selves from our "ill selves." Our everyday events are much more than joint ventures with our illness, but are a separate and very distinct part of who we are. When we are able to view our lives this way, we are free to discover ourselves without condition; we begin to dream again, we create ourselves anew. And as Dean so poignantly reminds us, a bit of humor and determination can go a long, long way in getting us there.

We can imagine life on Cripple Creek, because we glimpse ourselves on every page. These, too, are your challenges, your days in the life with multiple sclerosis. And like Dean, perhaps you will come to embrace the difficulties and laugh at the myriad of trials that life presents to us. You, with all your dreams and disappointments, can sit in the raspberry patch and remember the gift that life is, no matter its twists and turns. And somewhere near the last page, riding high above a field in Pennsylvania, I hope you too will embrace your own path. It's your road, after all; it's your Cripple Creek.

Margot Russell, author of *When the Road Turns*

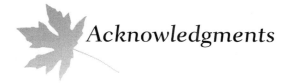 Acknowledgments

THERE ARE A GREAT MANY to whom I owe gratitude for help along the way. First, though, I want to offer thanks to God for the many blessings and challenges that grace my life. Next, I absolutely could not and would not have made this book without the enthusiasm of Margot Russell, my friend and agent. It was she who initially brought my essays into print in her own book, *When the Road Turns: Stories By and About People With Multiple Sclerosis*. Margot is the one who first suggested I might put together a book of my own. Ignoring my disbelieving hesitation, she found a publisher who enjoyed my work as much as she did, negotiated the project of which this book is the fruit, and put in long hours helping me organize and polish my effort. Margot makes dreams come true—even dreams one isn't aware of having.

I want to thank Dr. Diana M. Schneider of Demos Medical Publishing, Inc. She read my work with delight, appreciated its potential, and offered me a contract. Though admittedly I have no prior experience with which to compare, she seems to me the soul of cooperation, and I am grateful for all she's done.

I am also grateful to the staff and membership of MSWorld (*www.msworld.org*) for their support and encouragement from the start, especially Kathleen Wilson, Susan Zachary, and my online chat co-host and first editor, Yvon Sosville.

In addition to the above-mentioned colleagues there are friends, close and closer, whose caring and nurturing have furthered my progress as a writer. Among the closest of these is Susan Dudley, *aka* Twink, whose devoted companionship is truly a blessing. I deeply appreciate the welcome extended by Susan's family and the love of my old friend Sue Storey, who has stood in the role of surrogate parent to me since I was barely out of my teens. I offer thanks, too, to my mom and my sister for reconnecting with me and for never giving up.

I also want to thank Judith Waldman LCSW-C, A. Allan Genut, M.D., and Rev. Raymond B. Good. Each of them in differing, though not entirely dissimilar, ways has kept me well and each owns a share of my gratitude.

Finally, I want to thank each and every one of you who reads this book. Though we've never met, you've offered me this opportunity to connect with you, and that means a great deal to me.

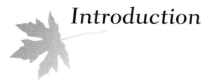

Introduction

Multiple Sclerosis (MS) is a disease of the brain and spinal cord. The disease is characterized by recurrent attacks of inflammation and the development of lesions in the white matter of the central nervous system, resulting in neurologic dysfunction. The attacks cause a wide variety of more or less disabling symptoms over time. The disability can be progressive. MS has no known cure.

I'VE ALWAYS BEEN A READER SO, when I finally accepted my neurologist's diagnosis of multiple sclerosis, I looked to the written material available to those of us with the disease. There were many medical resources with lists of symptoms and descriptions of available treatments. There were a few autobiographies by people with MS, which were, in the main, lists of their symptoms and descriptions of available treatments they'd undergone. There were testimonial books, in which people claimed to have cured themselves using various diets, spiritual practices, and other disciplines (although as yet no across-the-board cure has been found). There were articles about people who triumphed over the limitations imposed by the illness to perform some extreme feat such as mountain climbing, race-car driving, and the like. There were also compendiums of helpful tips for coping with the disabilities that one might eventually face with MS. But nowhere could I find what I wanted—books about the ongoing, everyday lives of ordinary people living with this disease. Nor at the time, with one exception, were there authors whose books described the gamut of emotional and spiritual (for lack of a better word) changes brought about within oneself through the experience of multiple sclerosis.

The exception was Nancy Mairs, an essayist whose book *Waist High in the World* described her myriad thoughts and feelings as she came to terms with MS. Taking Ms. Mairs as my inspiration, and with the cooperation of the staff at the MS support organization, *www.msworld.org*, I began writing essays detailing the everyday adventures, both internal and external, of my own ordinary life with MS. The essays appeared at MSWorld's web site on a monthly basis. I chose the title "Life on Cripple Creek" for several reasons. Most concretely, I live in a very rural area alongside a creek, I play the five-string banjo and "Cripple Creek" is a tune I love to pick, and, back in the late 1960s, early 1970s, a group called The Band did a song called "Up on Cripple Creek," that was a favorite of mine. More abstractly though, *cripple* is a word dear to my heart as one with MS and, although some may object to its use, I am, again, indebted to the work of Nancy Mairs for inviting me to consider it.

Contemplate the word *cripple*. It stands on its own without any modifiers. *Disabled* automatically calls *able* to mind as an opposite. *Differently abled* does the same. Those last two terms have the word "able" as their bottom line and then are modified with "dis" and "differently" so as to include the rest of us. But a cripple is beyond compare. Why, you'd have to say *not crippled* or *uncrippled* to get to an opposite. Imagine a world in which you needed some special verbal circumlocution to describe people as other than crippled. And there's another interesting aspect of this word *cripple*: there is no degree implied. How crippled is a *cripple*? Gloria Steinem, when she turned 50, was told, "Gee, you don't look 50." The reply attributed to her is, "This is what 50 looks like." When I use *cripple* to describe myself and someone responds, "Gee, you don't *look* crippled," I can paraphrase Ms. Steinem saying, "This is what *crippled* looks like."

I think about the words *Gay* and *Jewish*. Those are also descriptive words for groups of people—and words that stand on their own. Although both groups are minorities in this nation of, in large measure, heterosexual Christians, we don't refer to Gay people as *sexually disoriented* or to Jewish people as *differently spiritual*. So, what is it about a cripple that requires such careful language?

I have heard people object to the word *cripple* and, more recently, *MSer* for one who has MS because such labels limit a person. "I am more than my disease" people have said. When I call myself *crippled* I am speaking *in terms* of my disease. I call myself by other words at other times, as do we all. In other contexts I describe myself as *female, middle-aged, a writer* without finding those labels limiting or objectionable. When I perform a taxing physical feat and say, with grinning satisfaction, "Not bad for a crippled lady!" I definitely *mean* to be seen in the context of

3

my disease. To avoid all reference to such a reality or to go to lengths to disguise it is, to me, evidence of denial and a form of dishonesty.

Certain words, and we can all think of a few, were once used only pejoratively, as slurs, until the people so described took the words and empowered themselves by using them with pride. I propose to do the same with the word *cripple*, if only for myself. I certainly won't any longer be shamed out of using it to describe myself when I wish. It's an ancient and respectable word for a state of being in which, to some extent, I find myself.

So, with those ideas in mind, I gave my column at MSWorld its name. Shortly after it began to appear online, others with MS started writing to me of their own adventures, their own thoughts and dreams, and the changes wrought upon their lives by the disease. Even people *without* the disease wrote to share their struggles. I felt very blessed to be connecting with folks in this way.

It now seems to me that each of us has some crippling condition—physical, emotional, or spiritual, perhaps only situational—with which to come to terms. Each of us does this work with whatever gifts we've been given. I've been honored with the opportunity to offer this collection of essays. Whether or not you have multiple sclerosis or know someone who does, and no matter what word *you* like to use for people such as myself, I hope you will find something here to interest or amuse you and to accompany you on your journey. I thank you for taking the time to look into *Life on Cripple Creek*.

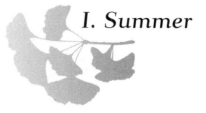

I. Summer

SUMMER IS A GREAT TIME to live on Cripple Creek. The fine weather allows nearby friends to be more available, while city friends look forward to a visit in the country. The beauty of the flowers, the bounty of wild fruits, and the cool depths of the pond are all attractions that keep me happily at home rather than wishing to be away.

But summer is also a difficult season for those with MS. The heat and humidity can cause nerves to misfire, just as overheating can short out an uninsulated wire. It's necessary for many of us to avoid long sojourns in the sun. To this end, after short forays outdoors, I spend much time inside in air-conditioned comfort.

The following four essays were written over several summers.

The Stress Paradox

ONE THING those of us with MS are often told by our doctors is that we should try to avoid stress. In other words, we should accept having an incurable neurologic disease that may or may not cripple us more or less completely (and who knows when?); and, while doing that, we should avoid feeling stress. We are told to go home to our parents, partner, and children, with this horrible news; go back to work being, perhaps, unable to *divulge* this horrible news; and (by the way) try to keep clear of stressful situations. Are you with me so far? We are offered incredibly expensive treatments that many of us cannot afford, which may or may not work (but there's nothing better out there)...and, meanwhile, try to keep a lid on stress, okay? Ummm, is it just me, or is there something just a hair of a tad *impossible* about this suggestion?

There's some evidence (and for many of us the experience) that MS symptoms worsen with stress. This is true for both physical and cognitive symptoms. The paradox is that, when under stress, we are *more* likely to need what there is *less* of, be it physical prowess or the ability to think. Here are two little illustrations from my own adventures...

One day in early summer, I rode my scooter near to our raspberry patch to pick some berries. I can ride any of several different paths mowed to that patch. The paths consist of narrow lanes with high brush on either side. I was feeling spry that day, so I dismounted part of the way there and walked down the path to the patch. As

I moved forward, picking, I stepped on a ground-hornets' nest. One of them stung me and others were coming out of the hole. I couldn't run at all. Running for me is *totally* no longer an option. I couldn't walk back to my scooter because the nest was between me and it. I couldn't force my way through the thick brush, either. All I could do was stagger along the path away from my scooter hoping to circle back to it on another lane. And I laughed as I staggered because the mental stress of being pursued by hornets was causing my legs to become like two sacks of wet cement. Laughing added to the physical stress I experienced. The more I laughed, the less well I staggered. The less well I staggered, the more I laughed. Toddling along as quickly as I could, I remembered the theory that bee stings alleviate MS symptoms, which made me laugh even harder. It's possible that the sound of maniacal laughter and a slow pace (as opposed to fleetness of foot and shrieks of fear) confused the hornets enough that they quit following me. At any rate, I was able to circle back to my scooter on another path and get home safely and relatively unharmed. The point is that I was in trouble, needed my legs, and yet could rely on them less than usual precisely because I needed them.

On another occasion, I was out shopping and returned to my car. My car has an automatic shift with the options P R N D D̲ 1 2. I was parked head-in and started the engine. But then I was stumped! There I sat, trying to remember whether I needed D or D̲ to back the car out of the space. I was sure that one "D" meant *drive forward* and the other meant *drive backward*, but for the life of me I couldn't think which was which. My brain had become stuck on the idea that I was going to "drive" the car, and therefore

I needed a *drive* gear. I became increasingly frustrated at my inability to remember, and the more frustrated I became, the less clearly I was able to think through the problem. I was aware enough of the potential for danger that I did not try to move the car until I'd figured out which gear-setting to use. As far as MS cognitive problems are concerned, the good news is that it isn't Alzheimer's disease. The bad news? One may *forget* that it isn't Alzheimer's disease. But, because it *isn't* Alzheimer's disease, one eventually remembers again. And in this case I eventually remembered again that I needed R for *reverse* rather than D or <u>D</u> for *drive*.

A few things have helped me with the MS stress paradox. One important lesson I've been teaching myself is that I don't have to be perfect, nor do I have to be exactly as I was before MS. When I can remind myself of this, I'm able to let go of the shame and the panic that often accompany an increase in impairment during times of stress. Releasing those useless feelings gives me a little more space to think a problem through. *That* enables me to solve some physical or mental predicaments more efficiently. I've begun to allow myself to be *slow*. Sometimes I want to take whatever time it takes to solve a problem for *myself* (as long as there's no danger) and, instead of asking for help or berating myself for being stupid or weak, I work my way through it at my own, cognitively impaired pace, and come up with a solution that takes MS into account.

Conversely, I'm also giving myself permission to need help from others. Now, if someone is present to help, I might ask for assistance instead of telling myself I'm smart enough or strong enough to work my way out of any situation.

Life on Cripple Creek

I work outdoors a lot here on Cripple Creek. In June, I got my tractor stuck on a hillside while mowing tall brush in a very tight area. This was a stressful situation for both the tractor and myself. Prior to MS, I'd have quickly figured out how to free the tractor from its predicament. Now, I had no clue. But I did not panic or feel ashamed of myself. Instead, I sat there calmly running the engine with my foot on the clutch until I'd burned up the transmission belt. Then, I got off the tractor and began to work out a solution that took my MS into account. I had time. There was no danger. The tractor wasn't going anywhere soon. I decided that if I could lift the mower deck and free the half-mowed thorn bushes lodged beneath it, I might get the tractor back to the barn. I could have done this with one hand before MS. With MS, I reasoned, it was going to take my entire arm and my back muscles, too. In consequence, I wrenched the muscles in both my arm and back holding up the mower deck. With my other hand I pulled at the thorny branches. I had no work gloves because, in my cognitive impairment, I'd forgotten to wear them and, given my physical impairment, I wasn't going to waste energy walking back to the house to get them. Thus, bloody-handed and sore of arm and back, I finally managed to get the tractor back to the barn where, using another of my new-found skills, *asking for help*, I called the repair service to come and fix it.

Yes, the MS stress paradox can be handled using simple skills which *anyone* can learn. Except, apparently, I need more practice. Maybe by next June.

The Pitfalls of Good Health: or, "Now that You're in Remission, Dear, Please Mow the Lawn."

So FAR, it's been a very stressful summer here on Cripple Creek. My long-time, elderly friend and guardian, Sue, had to be rushed to the hospital. What seemed at first to be a simple gall bladder problem turned out to be several kinds of cancer. This woman, many years my senior, took me in when I was a young person with no good family connection to speak of. She helped me get an education and offered me a home. In many ways—ways that count—Sue is my mother. When I was able-bodied, I took care of her gardens and lawn. I did much of her "grunt" work. She made provision for my care should my MS worsen, and she has helped me at times when my MS was bad enough to require expensive assistive devices. In addition to whatever she has provided me, we have lived here, in separate houses, on Cripple Creek for many years. We visit once or twice each day. We laugh together. We have wonderful conversations. We know each other very well. So, she is more than just a good friend, and the thought of losing her to a relatively early death (which seemed quite possible) was almost unbearable.

As if this crisis wasn't enough, Sue's blind dog, Sam, which had been left to board at the local veterinarian's kennel when we rushed to the hospital, developed an infection and required surgery and careful monitoring. Now, Sue and I are very close. But Sue and Sam are even closer. Sam is Sue's deepest spiritual connection. So, it was an incredibly difficult situation. In fact, as I read over what I've written, it begins to sound like a rather over-dramatized Country-and-Western song. Well, I'm happy to report that after several weeks in the hospital, and extensive surgery, my friend and her dog are both back home at last. Sue's condition was both operable and manageable with medications, and she can expect many more years of healthful life. Sam is in great shape, too (still blind, though).

If you are wondering what all of this has to do with MS, be patient. Here it comes.

During this troubling time, I found myself having to take on responsibilities I wasn't sure I had the physical strength or stamina to handle. There was driving back and forth to the hospital each day, a round trip of some 70 miles. I had to park and walk into and out of the hospital. I had to fetch and carry things to my friend. I had to take care of her cat and other aspects of her house-keeping, including some cleaning, while she was gone. I had to make all sorts of decisions and remember all sorts of new details under stressful circumstances. Before Sue came home, I had to rearrange and install some furniture so that she'd be able to live relatively independently while recovering. When she returned home she was instructed not to lift things weighing more than 5 pounds for the next month. She couldn't drive. So I continued to do her lifting and her driving. All of this came on top of my usual chores and responsibilities. For years, Sue had been the able-bodied one. Now, although I was the one with MS, I'd become the able-bodied one. It's all relative.

About a year ago, I began experiencing either a big-time remission or an actual improvement in my symptoms. Up until that time

I needed a wheelchair to go more than a little distance. As recently as the previous September I'd needed a scooter to get around outside. Yet here I was, this summer, walking with no stick, lifting, shoving furniture, running errands, thinking clearly, and remembering details. Certainly, I got tired doing all of this. There are still times when my usual symptoms increase in intensity. But I also felt vital and extremely grateful that I was able to do all that was necessary. I suffered no exacerbation as a result of my efforts and, in fact, held onto my gains during the change of season from spring to summer (which had been a time of exacerbation in past years).

Like many with MS, in the past I had wanted to do more than was good for me. Exhausting myself trying to make a contribution, I'd become much more symptomatic. Then I wouldn't have the strength or energy left to do the things I'd really *wanted* to do. So, I learned to set limits. I learned that if I did the housecleaning on Saturday morning, I'd have to pass on a trip to the mall in the afternoon. I learned to make choices and to give others choices as well ("Would you rather I help you with your onerous household task or go with you to the dog show?"). I trained myself to ignore people who intimated that I was using my MS to goof off. And most of my friends understood, accepted the situation, and stopped intimating.

Well, you know MS. Whatever you decide is true about you and your disease, it's going to change one way or another, sometimes before the words are out of your mouth. The bittersweet result of my return to a more able-bodied position is that I had more to do than ever, and I really couldn't say "no" as I'd trained myself to do.

So, on a really hot day in July, I found myself considering and then accepting a timidly proffered request to push (*push!*) a lawnmower at a friend's house, this exercise to be followed by a trip to a monastery for a worship service. I mowed almost the whole lawn. I even allowed myself to gripe a little about how hard I was working. Toward the end my feet were floppy, and I got a little dizzy on the turns, but for the most part it was just like old, pre-MS, times. A few hours later, I went to the service. It was a Catholic church and, what with genuflecting and so forth, I got plenty of exercise there, too. I was able to do both of these activities without having to choose between them. I began to rethink the whole idea of limits due to MS, as I was no longer sure what mine might be. What a wonderful thing to have to do!

So, all of you with MS who are putting energy into imagining a return to some sort of health, remember the saying "be careful what you ask for" (especially where friends' lawns are concerned); but, for *goodness* sake, don't quit asking!

Never Forget to Remember

THOSE OF US who have MS don't talk about cognitive impairment very openly, even among ourselves. For one thing, given that MS often doesn't progress until middle age, we usually begin to experience these problems at a time when many of our friends *without* MS are starting to speak of forgetfulness. Thus, we may not initially recognize our problems as MS-related. Then, too, any person with MS working hard to compensate for *physical* disability wants to believe she at least has full control of her *thought* processes. But cognitive impairment can be a very real part of the MS picture for some of us.

I have been struggling to write about this subject for quite a while. Writing is what I do, but *struggling* to write is a new experience for me. It's scary to be unable to think clearly—it's a very helpless feeling. When writing, I've noticed myself misspelling words more often. I have trouble with homonyms these days, using *their* when I really mean *they're*, for example. My computer's spell-checking program doesn't catch these errors since they are actual words rather than misspellings, making the situation particularly embarrassing when sending e-mail.

In my speech, I tend to mispronounce words that used to fall trippingly from my tongue. The other day I put way too many *esses* in speaking of the NMSS (National Multiple Sclerosis Society). I was speaking to an administrator of that organization, sounded as if I'd swallowed a *sssnake* and felt like a complete *assss*. Sometimes, when speaking, I forget a word and have to seek a suitable substitute in mid-sentence. The substitute I choose may be just off the mark, turning my utterance humorously incomprehensible. One day, unable to think of *impugn* I spoke of *impinging* someone's honesty. My style of speech can be somewhat pompous, and now I occasionally find myself speaking somewhat pompous nonsense. It feels awful when I notice this happening, but it's even more awful when I'm oblivious at the time only to realize later that I must have seemed a total idiot. Like Humpty Dumpty as realized in Lewis Carroll's *Alice* books, I've always believed it was a question of who's in charge—I or the word. Words have been my pleasure and I, who have enjoyed playing with them, now feel as if I'm being played with *by* them.

Cognitive deficits make themselves apparent in other areas as well. Some of us have difficulty organizing our activities efficiently, particularly when under stress (a time when the ability to organize efficiently may be *particularly* necessary). Short-term memory loss is another common symptom those with MS have mentioned as troublesome. Older people refer to these as "senior moments." You might go upstairs to fetch something and find you've forgotten what it was by the time you've climbed the stairs. I used to laugh at the idea of someone searching diligently but vainly about the house for his glasses only to discover them perched on his head. I actually considered this to be something of a myth until I did it myself. Fortunately, most MS symptoms come and go. For the majority of us they seldom become profoundly incapacitating, although one can feel pretty incapacitated when experiencing them.

The burgeoning population of elderly folk has afforded a wealth of commercial opportunity for the makers of various gadgets guaranteed to make one's Golden Years less taxing. For handling memory problems, resources range in technologic sophistication—from sticky notes to digital recording devices the size of a credit card. Naturally, no one has yet solved the problem of how to remember one is *using* any of these things. I once came across a sticky note reminding me to remove something from the refrigerator before it went bad. The sticky note was so old that *it* had gone bad and I'd prefer not to describe what I found in the refrigerator.

I'd begun accepting the experience of MS, coming to terms with losses of physical competence and skill. While there are many activities I miss, I'm finding other pleasures to replace them. I'm discovering that *bodily stillness* can be as mindful and engrossing for me as action was at one time. In addition, I'm beginning to understand that when cognitive deficits are in evidence, I may have to learn to appreciate *stillness of mind*—intellectual stillness. To sit outdoors here on Cripple Creek on a summer's day without thinking about anything in particular can be a peaceful and a rewardingly centering experience.

Returning from town, I rest on a bench in the shade outside my door for a time. I become aware of the sounds of birds calling, of livestock mooing or baaing. There are branches scraping and grasses swishing. I hear the air itself as it passes. There's the sound of a neighbor chopping wood for next winter. An airplane roars overhead. A township dump truck grinds its gears somewhere down the road. Two children are screaming angrily at each other from a nearby farm, while another neighbor is shooting his rifle and still another is endlessly revving the engine of his never satisfactorily tuned racing car. This is not so peaceful. I think I'll go inside. Where are my keys? Where did I put those *keys? Oh, come on!* I *know* they're here *somewhere!* I'll just put my glasses on and search through my purse. Where are my *glasses?*

Push Comes to Shove

SOMETIMES, much as I love the rural solitude of Cripple Creek, I enjoy venturing into the nearest big city for festivals, concerts, crafts shows—whatever. On these occasions, I've learned that the difference between a miserable time and a great time is a manual wheelchair.

I used to take no assistive device or, at most, a cane to events that required me to be on my feet for an extended period. Within an hour or so, my feet were dragging or flopping uselessly and I became tired, cranky, and no longer a pleasure to be with. My long-suffering friends would accommodatingly return home much earlier than they'd expected. Alternatively, they'd park me on a bench somewhere to be bored out of my gourd. I was very whiney in those days, and I was asked out less and less often.

Even though I could still walk moderate distances, I came to see that a wheelchair would allow me to relax and enjoy pout-free outings. I acquired a manual chair that I could push myself. I used my new chair for the first time at a crafts show with a friend and was delighted to find that she grew tired long before I did. The chair came with standard indoor tires. I soon replaced them with knobby tires, so that the chair would function on rougher surfaces. Its pneumatic tires were eventually given foam inserts so that maintaining air pressure would not be a nagging worry. I attached a back pack and a drink-holder to the chair. I bought a pair of black leather fingerless cycling gloves to keep my dainty mitts clean and callus-free. I felt quite the well-outfitted cripple.

On outings, I wheeled myself for as long as I could. I have good upper body strength, and I enjoyed learning a few of the more sedate sporty moves in my chair. Soon, I could make dramatic sudden turns or jiggle the chair back and forth in place (my new equivalent of impatiently bouncing on the balls of my feet). When I got tired of wheeling myself, I'd ask a friend to push. My friends were actually *pleased* to push my chair. Initially, this was probably out of relief that we could stay out as long as they wished. But over time, it became clear to me that there is something almost dangerously liberating about a wheelchair for the pusher as well as for the pushed. If I knew enough about psychiatric diagnosis, I'd be tempted to categorize people on the basis of their pushing styles.

I have one mild-mannered friend who was very insistent that she be allowed to push the chair. She wouldn't take *no* for an answer. She'd taken time to learn about MS and fatigue and wanted me to have a good time without overexerting myself. Unfortunately, she turned out to be incapable of remembering the foot-rests extending beyond the front of the wheelchair's seat. When we were in a crowd she invariably bumped me into the calves of the person in front of us. That person, naturally, turned around and glared—at *me*. I'd apologize, then turn around and glare at my *friend*, and she'd *giggle*.

"*Please!*" I begged her, "remember that my feet are sticking out down here. Try not to get too close to the people in front of us, okay?" She'd say she was sorry. She'd promise to be more careful. We'd wheel along for another few feet until *bam*, and she'd giggle again. I don't know what the problem was. She couldn't *see* my feet and *out of sight, out of mind*, I guess. I tried warning her as we approached those ahead, but it's hard to project your voice behind you and she said she couldn't hear me. I tried to stop the chair myself, reaching down and grabbing the rails, but instead of noticing where my hands were she viewed the resistance as an obstacle to be overcome and pushed harder, which resulted in more violent contact. This woman, reserved of affect and the type who wouldn't harm a fly, was soon giggling before we'd even hit the next hapless pedestrian. Something apprehensive in the set of my shoulders, seen from her perspective behind me as we approached, seemed to set her off. Now, upon impact, she'd burst into gales of helpless laughter. Toward the end of her tenure, I'd refuse to let her push. But I'd get tired, she'd plead, and I'd relent. Although she claimed to be trying for better awareness, we'd inevitably run into someone we didn't know. I finally had to fire her as a pusher because I was afraid someone would initiate a lawsuit.

Truth be told, had I paid attention to her driving style and put two and two together, I never would have permitted her to push me in the first place.

The next person to offer to push my chair is a very sweet, vegetarian, nonviolent, and spiritual woman—my companion, Twink. I have read that a woman who gets behind the wheel of an SUV undergoes a personality change that turns her from a safety-conscious, polite, and somewhat timid driver into a raging rhino of the raceway. I'm here to tell you (and thank God I *am* here to tell you) that the same phenomenon occurs when certain women get behind a wheelchair.

Twink, my chair, and I went to a very large, very crowded street festival celebrating the arts. There were concerts on several outdoor stages, crafts booths, art displayed along the sidewalk, installations of sculpture, and performance artists abounding, as well as foods of all kinds sold from wagons and tents. All this activity was crammed into a few blocks of one city street. Although I initially insisted I could wheel myself, the street rose uphill from the festival's starting point, and I quickly grew tired. Cheerful Twink offered to take over. This was her first experience with a "loaded" wheelchair. The chair is well-balanced, but Twink is a short, petite woman and at that time I outweighed her by 30 pounds. This festival is traditionally held on the hottest three days of the summer. Before long, my small friend was puffing and sweating. I told her I'd get out and walk (shades of pioneers' oxen-drawn wagons heading over Pike's Peak). She merrily insisted she was fine (she used to be a cheerleader) and continued pushing us to our destination—a band-shell where a friend was scheduled to perform.

Because I was in a wheelchair, I was permitted to park myself close to the stage and Twink was pleased to benefit from this situation. But our friend's band is a popular one. People began crowding around us. Then a few made the mistake of stepping in front of me. My own tendency in such cases is to politely ask the human obstructions to respect my need as a disabled person and, if they must stay in the disabled seating area, to avoid blocking my view. But Twink, with her hands on the wheelchair, spoke from her newfound position as my guardian and said something which began, *"Hey! Idiot!* Yeah, you, with the camera!"

I can't remember the rest of what she said because the next thing I knew, some unfortunate had dropped a still-burning cigarette butt on the ground by my chair. *"Yo!* Do you think the woman in this wheelchair wants to smell your *stinking tobacco?"* I couldn't quite grasp that this was the gentle, people-pleasing Twink of my past experience.

The day continued to unfold. We left the band-shell and went to one of the indoor art galleries. There was a strip across the threshold of the entrance to the gallery, and Twink was having a hard time with the chair. Finally, she looked at a bystander and with all the sarcasm she could muster said, *"Excuse me!* Do you think you could be *bothered* to lend a *hand* here?" After viewing the work inside, we made our way to the exit. Someone jumped with alacrity to hold the door. Did Twink offer a simple word of thanks? No, it was, "Thank you. That was very kind. At least *some* people know how to act."

We proceeded to the food area. There was a special tent with tables for physically disabled people to sit and eat. A board had been placed as a ramp leading up to the tent. Twink aimed my chair at the board and (had it been an SUV) *floored it.* The chair hit the board's raised edge and flung me forward. I saved myself a spill by grabbing the armrests. Twink continued ramming, muttering in frustration about the stupid incompetents who'd placed the board so uselessly. She was oblivious of my suggestion that she tilt the chair. She refused to let me get out and walk. "You shouldn't *have* to walk. Don't these people know how to set up a ramp?!" I managed to keep my seat until, finally, some Good Samaritan helped her lift the chair onto the ramp. We rolled up to the tables, which were filled with able-bodied people unaccompanied by cripples. To them, the empty tent with tables must have looked like a cool, shaded place to eat—respite from the press of the crowd. Twink glared at these people in disgust. *"Clear out!"* she commanded, "This is *handicapped* seating! Do any of *you* have a handicap? I don't *think* so." The diners looked her over, saw the glint in her eyes, the set of her jaw, and her fists on her hips. With sheepish expressions and in silence they packed up their meals and left.

I'm not intensely outspoken politically when it comes to the rights of the disabled. I've tended to talk softly when I felt I must and to keep silent more often than is, perhaps, wise. Although I'd been hunched in my chair with embarrassment during each of these interactions, I was beginning to note the way folks jumped when Twink said, *"Jump!"*

Our meal over, we headed back to the car. We were now going down the long hill up which Twink had valiantly pushed me earlier that day. We were marching in lock-step due to the numbers of people around us, and I could sense her impatience at the slow pace. At one point, a woman and her husband cut directly in front of us and Twink, braking suddenly to avoid hitting them, said "Hey! Watch where you're going! I've got a *disabled person* here. Try looking below *eye-level* sometime!" The woman glared—at *me*, of course, and angrily started to say something, but her husband grabbed her and hauled her off into the crowd. This event had cleared a little space around us and Twink walked more quickly with the chair. She trotted, and then broke into a run. People dodged left and right. Twink bellowed, *"Out of the way! Disabled person coming through!"* Our momentum increased, and I realized Twink was no longer pushing the chair—she was simply hanging on to it or even being pulled by it. Was I terrified? Yep.

But as our descent continued, I began to feel exhilarated. I enjoyed the cooling breeze in my hair. I was used to people sighing in irritation over having to make room for my chair. I was used to having to request passage, ignored by those who chose not to "see" me. Now I grinned at the novelty of people fleeing for their lives. *"Whooeee!"* we yelled, *"Yip! Yip! Yip!"* We were flying!

At the bottom of the hill, Twink brought the chair to a halt, told me how much fun she was having, and told me *I* was having fun, too. I agreed. We met some friends we knew and stopped to talk with them. I stood up from my chair for this. A pleasant and convivial exchange ensued when along came the couple Twink and I had almost hit at the top of the hill. The woman saw me standing there and turned to her husband, "See?" she said, "That woman isn't even disabled! Look at her standing there. Where do people get off!" While my response to her was a smile and a wave, this was the last straw for Twink.

"Have you ever heard of *multiple sclerosis?*" she began, her volume increasing as she stalked toward the woman, *"Do you have any idea what that IS? Do you have ANY IDEA what it's like to have a neurologic disease?"* Again, the woman's husband took her arm and they disappeared into the surging mass of humanity as Twink continued shouting after them, *"What is your PROBLEM? Do you ever think of anyone besides YOURSELF?!"* In her empowered righteousness she was a wonder to behold. Our friends stared at her in awe.

I've come further into remission since that last outing in my chair. I still take my wheelchair on day trips, but I don't always ride in it. Instead, I use it as a walker, pushing it myself from behind. The seat provides a handy place for storing purchases, and I can still sit and use it a bit if I get too tired to walk. People look at me askance as I push an empty wheelchair. I don't mind the quizzical looks. They are a relief, actually, because they hold no potential for shouting-matches, lawsuits, or bodily injury. I am grateful not to be a catalyst for the character defects of my friends, now that it is my good fortune to be able to walk in contented safety. If you are able-bodied and attend the same events as I, it is *your* good fortune as well.

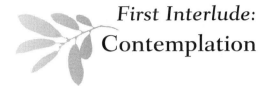

First Interlude:
Contemplation

THE NEXT FIVE ESSAYS all have in common an underlying concern with thoughts about identity given MS. When I first came to Cripple Creek I lived alone. I was coming to terms with past difficulties and spent much of my time in meditation as I wandered the woods and fields. I tried to connect with what I choose to call God. Even though I now share my life more intimately with others, I still make time to reconnect with that which I conceive to be greater than myself each day. As it once helped me handle solitude, such time now helps me with the challenges of living with another.

In addition, MS offers its own challenges on many levels, mental as well as the more obvious physical ones. MS can affect my ability to think, when cognitive symptoms are present. It has also deeply influenced my experience of myself and the world around me, changing my perceptions of both over time.

Who Do I Think I Am ?

A WHILE AGO I read a book by Israel Rosenfield called *The Strange, Familiar and Forgotten.* Dr. Rosenfield, a neurologist, describes his book as "an anatomy of consciousness." His basic thesis—and this is a grand oversimplification on my part— is that one's self-awareness grows neurologically from, and is nurtured by, one's physical existence. The feedback between these two states begins in infancy and continues throughout one's life. Furthermore, consciousness is not a static state, but is *dynamic*, changing with the vicissitudes of one's neurology and experience. I thought it a pretty apt book for a person with MS to be reading, since such a person's neurologic experience can change from one hour to the next.

I consider who I thought I was before MS, versus who I think I am now. Those of us who have MS talk at times of the work we used to do, relationships we used to have, activities we once enjoyed. Sometimes we sound as if we feel we've now lost validity as people. It's as if we're saying, "Hey! I wasn't always a cripple! I was a (fill in the blanks): retail buyer, husband, skier. I was *somebody*." If we took our sense of self from those jobs, connections, or pastimes, and have since lost them, we may be unsure of who we are within the context of MS.

I often tell people that I am much improved through having MS—am a much "better" person than I was in the days when I took neurologic health for granted. Other folks with MS from whom I've heard have expressed similar feelings. They've put it in terms of understanding the sufferings of others more fully than they used to. When I say I'm a "better" person now, I'm talking about something more profound than a changed viewpoint. I'm talking about a total "rewiring of self" (which, indeed, is no metaphor). For example, when I could move quickly, efficiently, and gracefully, I was often counseled by my elders to slow down, learn stillness, practice patience. And I wanted to do those things, so I tried to do them as I was then—quickly, efficiently, and gracefully. But MS has *recreated* me as a slow-moving, physically inefficient, and clumsy person, and, in gifting me with stillness, has required both patience and acceptance. Although I did not develop these qualities through an effort of will, I am surprised and pleased to find myself experiencing them.

MS gives different gifts to each of us. I know of those with MS who, formerly content, have been gifted with frustration. Some of these people do not in the least welcome this gift. But many are using it to fight discrimination against the disabled and to improve the quality of life for others, because the gift of frustration has increased their discomfort and awareness in those areas. Others are using frustration to find creative solutions to daily tasks that they can no longer accomplish as they once did. Conversely, my gifts of patience and acceptance have allowed me to give *up* doing some of the things I used to think absolutely *had* to be done.

These new qualities, these gifts of MS, whether or not one enjoys them, become one's experience of who-I-am. And one is challenged to come to terms, not just with physical limitations, but with an *identity* arising from one's brand new (and ever-changing) body. I think about all of this as I ride my scooter beside Cripple Creek. I would never have chosen to have this disease, and I look forward to a cure. But in its way, MS has asked me "Who do you think you are?" And it's challenged me to engage in an ongoing, dynamic dialogue with my own neurology. For these simple but profound gifts, I am truly thankful.

Out of My Mind

I SOMETIMES TEND to overdo it, as many with MS do, never sure of my limits. I was influenced early in life by old "Romper Room" TV shows, and I still long to be a good do-bee and not a bad don't-bee. I suppose this attitude ought not surprise me. Our society rewards competitive striving with material success and marginalizes those who cannot compete. I've been exposed to society's drive-and-strive values my whole life, and in all that time no one prepared me for the tellingly termed unthinkable—a disabling condition. I live with others on Cripple Creek and, as regards activity levels, I want what's best for both myself and my family. It's hard to find that balance among the uncertainties of MS. What's "best" now may not be "best" in an hour. With its many unknowns, mostly beyond my control, MS leaves the door open for moral judgments that wreak havoc on my self-esteem. I get caught between my desire to be lauded a winner who can just do it and my fear of condemnation as a loser who, unable to run with the big dogs, must stay on the porch. The result of this conflict is that, regardless the opinions of others, I hand myself the most damaging judgments from within, sentencing myself to life in a prison of my own creation for the crime of not knowing when enough is enough.

I have a friend whose mother sensed an impending heart attack and drove several miles out of her way to return some library books on the due date before checking into a hospital. When I heard this story, I thought the woman was *nuts*. But often, feeling the need to sit and rest, I force myself to do *one last thing* out of fear I might otherwise be a slacker. An example—finished with work for the day, I haul myself wearily upstairs for a snooze. "*Uh-oh,*" I say, glancing at the stair treads, "*dog hair. This ought to be swept.*" I decide that although I may *want* to lie down, I don't really *need* to yet. I can do this *one last thing*, and I head right back down the stairs for the broom and dust pan. This is sanity, right?

While in remission, I suffer the delusion that by doing as much as possible *today*, I can compensate for the day when I am no longer able to do much of anything. I buzz, a demented *do-bee*, driving myself to exhaustion. I get the groceries in, the laundry done, the clothes folded, the floors vacuumed, the counters wiped down, the dog-yard messes scooped, and the toilet bowl (*for Pete's sake*) cleaned, and why? *In case I end up in a wheelchair someday!* If I do all this work *now*, no one can *then* call me lazy. Does that make sense? And after putting myself through this marathon of maintenance, I wait in impatient expectancy for others to show appreciation for all I've done. You couldn't call the house clean, either, because it's now filled with *resentment*—both mine and that of my family members.

No longer living alone, I have not learned how to pace myself. I binge on *doing* and then flip-flop into a self-protective refusal to budge. I tell myself that unless I keep up the pace, I'm useless. Then I feel overwhelmed by all I've committed to doing. I worry that others may feel manipulated by my handling of MS. No worries there! How could they not?

Fortunately, before (or shortly after) driving those around me to distraction, I've realized that the negative running commentary of my Inner Prosecuting Attorney is dangerous to my well-being.

Although I'd learned to handle my limitations while living alone, I'm now having to learn to accept and respect them while living in constant comparison with an able-bodied person. It's a relatively new situation and, consequently, I've been experimenting with some new ideas.

I've been paying more attention to the language I use. Take the words *one last thing*. I've always been somewhat concrete in my thinking. These days, I try to think of those words literally. If I'm too tired to sweep the dog hair from the stair treads, yet feel driven to do so, I might imagine my family gathered solemnly outside my room in the hospital. The doctor has just delivered the worst possible news. Faces fill with grief. There are tears. Then someone quietly remarks, *"Well, at least she left the stair treads clean and free of dog hair."* The rest of them give approving nods. This thought wakes me up. As long as I live, there will be *one last thing* to do (and it will, most likely, involve dog hair). I can choose to pass on the sweeping once in a while.

I'm trying not to trap myself by asking whether I *need* a rest or merely *want* one. The English language differentiates those words and considers *need* the more acceptable of the two. Other languages have but one word, *will* (as in the sentence, *I will that it be so*) covering both concepts. It's relaxing to *will* myself a rest, no longer torn with anxiety between valid *need* and frivolous *want*.

As for the Manic Housework Martyr, I've come to see that others in my home have their own priorities for the use of my energy. Perhaps someone is willing to forego folded laundry if I'll go along on an errand. Others (with four legs and fur) would probably enjoy some time outdoors with me more than a vacuumed rug. People in good health need not choose among activities to such an extent, but I'll have to continue making choices as I ride the tide of relapse and remission with a loved one in my life just as I did when there was no such comfort. I've found that it furthers intimacy in very rewarding ways when I listen to the *true* needs of others, rather than projecting my own fears of incompetence and then trying to compensate. Instead of assuming, I'm becoming both more obser-vant and more likely to ask those with whom I live to help me choose which contributions they'd appreciate from me.

Naturally there will still be times when I judge my limited abil-ities poorly and sentence myself to doing more than I can handle. There will also be times when I feel imprisoned by the misun-derstanding of others regarding my MS. It's been written, *bars do not a prison make*. Bars may not, but minds certainly can. I'm try-ing to keep mine open.

Chicken Little and The Terminator

THERE'S A DIFFERENCE between an MS *flare-up* (an increase in old symptoms, usually limited in scope and duration), and an exacerbation or *attack*, (usually lasting longer and involving *new* symptoms, as well as an increase in old ones). As regards my own experience, I'm never sure at the outset which is which because it can take several days to resolve into one or the other. Everyone has good days and not-so-good days. But with MS, the potential always exists for the bad days to be a prelude to more serious disability. We are given all sorts of reasonable advice on how to reduce the likelihood of this occurring: take prescribed medications regularly, avoid overdoing it physically, lead a low-stress life, get good nourishment and enough sleep. I've also been offered advice that strikes me as not quite reasonable: don't wear lavender, do spend time under a pyramid, don't eat certain foods during certain phases of the moon. But, in truth, no one can predict the course of this disease with complete assurance in anyone's particular case.

I used to become frightened by the slightest intensifying of my symptoms. *"The MS is getting worse! The MS is getting worse!"* shrieked the voice of my Chicken Little-within, whenever my symptoms seemed more prevalent. My mind scrambled frantically, trying to ascertain what I might have done to bring this on. Had I been regularly taking my medications? Had I eaten a surfeit of mangoes during the full moon? Did I carry too many loads of laundry up the stairs? And, more importantly, I wondered what I could do to arrest it. Should I disengage socially? Did I need more sleep? Ought I to try the latest nutritional fad? Of course, I didn't display this panic to anyone. Like many with MS, I try to have a positive attitude, showing the world my *game face*. Thus, if friends noticed my fatigue or increased spasticity and asked concerned questions, I reassured them in the confident, laconic tones of my Terminator persona, "No problem" and "I'll be back!"

When my MS first became symptomatic on a regular basis, much of my conflict in living with it resulted from the differences between these two internalized characters. The Terminator was the one who attempted to carry luggage and move furniture, whereas Chicken Little nagged about the potential danger in such activities. After a busy day, Chicken Little thought we'd best stay home and watch the tube, while the Terminator made arrangements to go food shopping.

In my imagination, everyone, among them my friends and family, liked the Terminator better. I liked the Terminator better, too. In that guise, I was strong and could get things done. I didn't slow anybody down, wimp out, or cancel plans at the last minute. Say someone on Cripple Creek needed a hand getting a load of lumber onto the pick-up truck. Even though they'd say, "Oh, I don't want to ask YOU to help. You have MS. It will be too much for you," there was a weary shading in their tone of voice which suggested that they really wished I could just get over this MS nonsense and give them a hand. Naturally I wished this, too, and so...

"No problem," the Terminator would respond, "I will help." I would even go so far as to offer to do the job *all by myself*, leaving the person free for other tasks. In Terminator mode I was a *hero*, by golly! I felt more useful, more in control, and less at the mercy of my disease. As regards MS, perceiving myself to be in charge was a delightful fantasy to indulge.

On the other hand, Chicken Little was a misapprehending fool. She ran about in fear of an event that wasn't even happening and, in her conviction, caused her friends to fear as well. When I began to have difficulty walking, did Chicken Little advise me to purchase a cane and get on with my life? No. In a panic, (*"the MS is getting worse!"*) Chicken Little totally rearranged my kitchen so that everything would be accessible from the wheelchair she was convinced lay in my immediate future. When I needed to change from a car with a standard clutch to an automatic shift, Chicken Little had me buy a car with, in addition to the automatic transmission, a ramp and *hand-controls!* Under her direction, I learned to use many other assistive appliances which, to this day, I do not yet truly need. My Chicken Little qualities spread panic among my friends and family, causing them to become frightened for and more protective of me. Then the Terminator would step up and dismiss their concerns, leaving them baffled and, perhaps, mistrustful. And all I had to say to them was, "You think *you're* baffled and mistrustful?? Try being *me!*"

Many of us with MS have been given this advice: *contact your doctor if you have new symptoms, or old symptoms that increase in intensity, for more than 48 hours.* But each of us is different and, after a number of flare-ups and at least two exacerbations over the years, I'm now able to distinguish between those types of events—the vicissitudes of MS, in my particular case. Flare-ups are far more common, more likely. My flare-ups seem to be a direct result of overdoing it. Even before MS, I was slow to react both mentally and physically. I tend to experience things in a delayed sort of way. Contrary to the opinions of many doctors, it can take my flare-ups a little over a week to resolve, so I need more than 48 hours to determine whether I'm in trouble or not. I continue an active life but, during a flare-up, am inclined to tell the Terminator to sit down, refusing some of the more grandiose physical challenges I and others would have me accept. At the same time, although I pay attention to my need for rest when flare-ups occur, I ask Chicken Little to shut up, and I no longer project a few bad days into a lifetime's incapacitation. I haven't had a serious attack in several years but, if awareness can overcome denial, I ought to be able to recognize one quickly enough. None of this is an exact science, mind you. And the disease is so personal—such an individual experience that—although I wish someone had taught me to distinguish *flare-up* from *attack* earlier in my life with MS, it's probably one of those things each of us must learn for herself.

As time goes by, I'm becoming a better negotiator in the ongoing conflict between Chicken Little and the Terminator, quieting the inner voices that used to push me to extremes. These days, invited to describe myself as a character from Storyland (which, actually, never happens but if it did), I'd opt for The Little Engine That Sometimes Could and Other Times Could Not. If you haven't read that one, that's because it's still being written.

Who's the Dummy?

It's not that I used to think of myself as "the sharpest tool in the shed," to quote the ogre in the movie *Shrek*, but I knew my brain worked pretty well. All through my school years and into my working life, I was viewed as someone who could be relied on to organize things sensibly and to remember details. I had great faith in my intellect and derived a large measure of my self-esteem from applying it. Encouraged to take my abilities very seriously, I developed an impatience toward those who couldn't see my way of approaching any task as the *Absolute and Totally Correct One*. I didn't mean to be cruel, but I used my mind as a skilled athlete uses her body, and others were intimidated. When choosing between the needs of a project versus the needs of the *people involved* in the project, I could be somewhat lacking in personal warmth and consideration. The reason I know of these unflattering assessments is that MS has so changed me that people are no longer intimidated and have become willing to tell me exactly how I came across back then. They are even beginning to laugh at me. I am even beginning to laugh at myself.

Here's an example of how seriously I used to take my intellect. A friend was teaching me to play contract bridge. There are two teams of partners in bridge and they bid for a contract. The person who wins the contract, plays his own hand and also that of his partner as a *dummy-hand*. The partner, or *dummy*, who isn't play-ing her own hand is encouraged to replenish the snacks and drinks that were to me a major attraction of bridge. In our little practice session, my friend and I played as partners. She won the contract and asked me, "If I won the contract, who's the dummy?" I was incensed!

"Dummy? *Dummy?*" I bellowed, "Are you implying that, because I lost the contract, I'm *stupid*?? Why, I'm just *learning* the game! What do you expect?" It took her a few tense minutes to interrupt this rant and draw my attention to the bridge terms she'd just spent the past half hour teaching me.

Although only recently explored in the literature surrounding the disease, MS can affect both cognition and emotion, depending on where in the brain demyelination occurs. Some people experience mood swings or depression, due not only to the stress of having MS but sometimes as a result of disease activity in the part of the brain where affect is influenced. Others of us experience short-term memory difficulties, trouble keeping details organized, and a reduced ability to process information quickly. If one had these abilities to any great extent to begin with, as I did, losing them can be a very useful and enlightening experience.

My memory is no longer reliable. Initially, I wasn't aware of forgetting things. They were simply forgotten. But after a few people had to remind me (*me!*) of details I'd have never let slip in the past, feelings of shame and embarrassment made me more careful. I began making lists. Unfortunately, the things I continued to forget never made it onto the lists, or the lists got misplaced and I couldn't remember where I'd put them. Then, too, I'd often forget my reading glasses, leaving me unable to read a list when necessary, assuming I'd remembered to bring it in the first place.

There were other signs of MS in my thinking. I was once a master at organizing space, whether moving a household or filling luggage for a trip. As with other symptoms in relapsing/remitting MS, cognitive symptoms come and go. You can't rely on an ability being present, or being gone, from one moment to the next. One *bad brain day,* I used my van to help a friend move house. While I was able to make a contribution, loading and distributing boxes, I certainly did not evince my former efficiency and, as a consequence, my suggestions were not the *Absolute and Totally Correct Ones* as would have been my experience before MS. I had to acknowledge, and did so with some difficulty, that my friend's suggestions were more apt than my own.

It took a while for me to own up to these deficits. Naturally, I didn't *want* to perceive them. I didn't want to believe that friends and family were correct in pointing them out. The deficits *themselves* may have stood in the way of my noticing to some extent (I had trouble remembering that I was having trouble remembering). I already mentioned the shame I felt once I became aware of the slips and glitches. As I grew more accustomed to the situation, shame was replaced by irritation with myself for not overcoming the situation. Recently those feelings have given way to another, more pleasant, one…

I was driving Twink into town from Cripple Creek. Despite a lack of familiarity with our exact destination, before MS, I'd have been able to plan our route. Based on my years of city-driving experience, the route I chose would have been *Absolutely and Totally Correct*. This time, feeling my brain not up to the task, I simply asked directions of Twink. I had forgotten we had a stop to make on the way. Twink reminded me, affectionately adding, "We're not the brightest bulb in the chandelier today, are we?" And instead of defending myself by finding fault with her, or covering my resentment and forcing myself to laugh along, instead of being embarrassed, I felt a burden lifted from me and, as it lifted, I chuckled with genuine amusement. I'd always believed I had to be correct all the time, intellectually quicker than others, completely focused on my own efficiency. Up until that moment in the car, I had no idea of the pressure I'd felt, all my life, to uphold my own self-imposed standard of intellectual excellence.

Whether our symptoms are primarily physical, cognitive, or a combination of both, MS takes something away from each of us. Whatever our abilities were before MS, they are certain to be influenced by the disease, to some extent, at some point. But if the disease strips you of a skill, it can also strip you of the competitiveness that is often bound up with *excellence* at a skill. I still feel embarrassed from time to time, and I certainly have moments of frustration with myself when my symptoms interfere, but I've written before that MS has made me a better person, and one way it's done so is by offering me the opportunity to shift from a competitive to a cooperative point of view. That shift leaves me much more open to and accepting of the realities of people other than myself. Beyond acceptance lies appreciation.

When the ogre described himself in song during the opening moments of *Shrek*, he wasn't putting himself down at all. He was singing with clarity and comfortable self-acceptance, *"I'm not the sharpest tool in the shed."* Neither am I (and likely never was). It's quite a relief.

The Dreamer

WHEN I WAS VERY YOUNG, I had frightening dreams in which I found myself flying through the air. I wasn't able to control my flight, however, and I'd rise higher and higher or else awaken while plunging speedily to certain death. As time passed, and I aged, I became more skilled in my dreams of flying. Eventually, I was able to *choose* to fly in dreams. I'd leap effortlessly into the air, propelling myself with my arms, frog-kicking my legs for momentum as in water. The angle of my torso determined the height of my flight. No longer frightened, I found these dreams exhilarating. Sometimes I flew to escape dangerous pursuit or to impress an audience. And *sometimes* it seemed that my own bubbling joy simply lifted me off my feet.

Another recurring theme in my dreams involved my having to negotiate architecture apparently designed by Rube Goldberg and Escher working as a team. Of particular difficulty in these dreams were the staircases that wound into eternity and bent back on themselves. They were always made of some flimsy material and often had treacherous moving parts. In these dreams, I wasn't able to fly and had to clamber and climb, risking a fall. Defeated by these buildings in my childhood, I became competent at negotiating such obstacles in my dream-life as a young adult. Eventually, I was even able to enjoy them as physically challenging problems to solve, no longer made anxious by them.

Over the years, I began to fly less and less often in my dreams, and I encountered fewer and fewer multidimensional staircases. My dreams became very pedestrian—literally. I walked, I ran, I used the strength of my body as it was in waking life. Sometimes I walked as astronauts are seen to on the moon, a vestige of my former flights. I no longer had the satisfaction of conquering tangled stairs.

At some point during these more settled years of dreaming, I was diagnosed with MS. Like many people with the relapsing /remitting form, I recovered from the first attack with no residual symptoms. Both awake and in my dreams, I continued to move as I always had. But eventually, the disease returned and affected my gait, balance, and coordination. It did *not*, however, affect my dreams. My dreaming mind didn't realize I had MS, even though my waking mind had accepted the situation. I still walked, ran, and used my strength, taking these abilities as much for granted in dreams now as I had once in waking life.

I remember clearly the first time I had MS in a dream. I was supposed to walk somewhere with a group and I had to decline because, I told them, *I have MS and can't walk that far.* As I dreamed this conversation, I noted with surprise that it was true! I really *did* have MS, along with the limitations it had imposed on my body in waking life.

Slowly, but steadily, my dreams have begun to feature the influence of MS. Sometimes I have a cane or use my wheelchair. Numb fingers have made their appearance, interfering with manual dexterity. Although in past dreams, when driving, my vehicle was nondescript, these days I drive my ramp-van. My dreams are becoming less physical, more conversational or descriptive. True, I missed flying when it left my dream-mind, but as I'd never flown in actuality, it wasn't a very *great* loss. I understand how acceptance of reality percolates down through the conscious mind and into the subconscious. I'm aware that healthy self-integrity must, for me, include MS. I've truly missed and mourned moving as my former able-bodied self in waking life. Now I've begun to grieve that loss in my dreams as well.

Still, in dreams, I sometimes have the incredibly gratifying experience of being able to move as I did before MS had its way. I don't take such dreams for granted anymore. Insofar as my lucidity while asleep allows, I revel. I have dreams in which I run with a grace that is long gone, and in them I no longer care whether I'm running toward something wonderful or away from something awful. I'm *running*. There are dreams in which I still possess the strength and athleticism to meet physical challenges. I don't worry about succeeding in these dreams. I just enjoy moving, bending, lifting, and climbing. And on some wondrously blessed mornings, I awaken with the lovely sensation of having gone dancing.

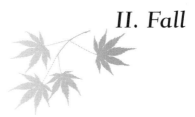

II. Fall

Autumn on Cripple Creek, with the trees in red and gold—a harvest-feast for the eyes. I ride my scooter around the pond and watch as day by day the water takes on a more wintry appearance, the geese and their fledged goslings head south, and the fish no longer jump in still afternoons.

With the cooler temperatures, I feel a renewed vigor. My ongoing symptoms seem to abate with the passing of summer's heat. There are lots of fall chores—cleaning up the garden, putting away the tractor, winterizing the windows—so I'm grateful to be less symptomatic.

Each of the next essays was written between summer's end and winter's arrival.

Everyday Heroes

ONE AUTUMN DAY, my friend Twink needed to respond to her elderly father's request that his two bulky, amazingly heavy reclining chairs be moved from the second to the first floor of the house where he lives.

In my imagination, here is how reclining chairs are manufactured: A frame of steel I-beams is encased in solid lead and the whole structure is then cast in concrete. This object is chiseled and sand-blasted into the shape of a chair. Holes are drilled and levers and springs are installed, whose major function is to pinch fingers. Secondarily, they cause the chair to recline, often at inopportune moments. The entire object is then padded and, finally, covered with a material which, no matter what it was initially, will degenerate into a filthy brownish-green substance related to fine upholstery only in Martha Stewart's worst nightmares.

Twink hired a very strong young man. Although we were willing to help, he was sure he could do the job on his own. "This will be no problem! Stand back, ladies," he said. He then single-handedly (a figure of speech if ever there was one) maneuvered each of these chairs out of the room they were in, through a hall, down a staircase, and into the living room where her father wished them placed. The maneuvering, (accompanied by such reassuring exclamations as *"Whoops!"* and *"Uh-oh!"*) included bashing (and then removing) a door, crunching (and subsequently replacing) a railing, and denting (and later repairing) some decorative woodwork.

A few days after this, dear old Dad decided he'd made a mistake. As cooler weather approached, he now wanted only *one* chair in the living room. The other recliner was to be returned to the warmer, more fuel-efficient room upstairs.

Among the celebrated heroes of disability offered us by the media are some who have accomplished feats requiring great physical courage, such as climbing a mountain, riding a bicycle across the desert, or competing in a triathlon. I am grateful to the pharmaceutical companies who feature such people in advertisements. They can inspire us and fill us with admiration for disabled people who realize their dreams however far-fetched they may seem—contending against all odds to achieve goals that, to the able-bodied, may seem foolhardy or way out of reach.

Foolhardy as it may seem to those of you with MS, I decided that Twink and I ought to be able to move *half* of what one person had moved by himself. We began our adventure with confidence and in high spirits, but in short order we found ourselves in dire circumstances. She was halfway up the staircase pulling on the upper back of the chair. I was at the bottom of the staircase supporting the weight of the chair and pushing. The recliner, stuck like a cork in a bottle, was wedged tightly between the railing and the opposite wall. We heaved at the chair but it went nowhere. As most mature people do when confronted with the need for cooperation in problem-solving, we began to argue over whose fault it was that the chair was stuck. Our tempers flared, as did my MS fatigue, and I knew time was running out for me. In desperate frustration, we gave the chair one last heave. The part she was holding suddenly flopped toward her almost pitching her down the stairs head first. The part I was holding suddenly lunged at me, punching me in the breadbasket. Apparently, during our final push the lever had caught on the railing and caused the chair to abruptly "recline." This was a very difficult situation and, as I often do in difficult situations, I began to laugh. If you have MS and ever find yourself beginning to laugh while wrestling with the business end of a recliner on a staircase, you'd better hope that, unlike me, urinary incontinence is *not* one of your symptoms.

Yes, we were finally able to get the chair back to its original room on the second floor and, yes, we are still friends (although neither of us is fond of her father at the moment). In fact, we are closer than ever, the result of surviving a grueling physical challenge. We learned we could trust each other when the going got tough. I also learned that, eyes blinded by tears from my insane cackling, I could climb over a reclining chair stuck on a staircase and get to the bathroom in record time.

The triumph I felt when we'd achieved our objective made me wish that, in addition to the wonderfully inspiring ads we're already offered, the companies that supply therapies for MS would also create ads featuring people who perform heroically in the more mundane activities of everyday life. One such ad might be headlined "Back to School" and could feature a mother with MS who, despite pain, fatigue, and cognitive short-circuiting, manages to get her three kids off to school on time that first important morning. She could be shown in her powerchair, fists raised in victory, the remains and wreckage of breakfast for three strewn about her kitchen. There would be a school bus in soft focus outside the window behind her. There's an ad I'd love to see!

The Jacket

AUTUMN IS HERE, winter is right on its heels, and I've been auditioning jackets again. I've auditioned several so far, and none of them has had a call-back. Last winter, I went through the entire season trying out coats for a few days at a time and then returning them as unsuitable. I never bought one to keep. Why all the difficulty? Well, the fault lies with MS, of course.

Multiple sclerosis isn't a static disease. You have the best of times, and you have the worst of times—along with all the times in between. So, I need a coat to cover several contingencies. It has to be comfortable in a wheelchair or on my scooter, yet cut well enough to look good when I can walk. It needs to be warm enough so that when I am moving quickly through the wind on my scooter I won't freeze, but not so warm that I will overheat when I am walking. I'm somewhat uncoordinated and weak, so my coat has to slide easily onto and off of the car's upholstered seats, and it can't add significantly to the weight I must carry. (If I get tired carrying the coat in its box from the UPS man's arms to my door, it's too heavy). I must purchase a coat from a catalog since shopping for clothing is very tiring, and I'm awfully clumsy in a dressing-room. At home, I can take my time and, if I stumble and ram my elbow through a flimsy partition wall, at least it's a wall I own.

I walk like a person who's had too much to drink—either too much alcohol, as when I stagger, or too much liquid, period, as when I am staggering quickly to a public restroom with my neurogenic bladder. So, it's important to me to look as smooth and well put-together as I possibly can. Whatever coat I choose must help me compensate for some of the dignity of which MS has robbed me.

Special coats for people in wheelchairs are designed to be worn when you're seated; they minimize both the bulkiness in your lap and the discomfort of being choked when you sit on your coat-hem. But that model won't work for me when I'm standing up. There are coats with double storm-flaps, and a multitude of pockets—Velcro-fastened pockets, snapped pockets, buttoned pockets. Most of these pockets are not easily accessed when seated. So, that won't work for me when I'm sitting down. And let me elaborate on closures...

I ride a scooter with throttle levers. One day, I went across the yard to visit my elderly friend Sue, whose house is next door to mine. She saw me from her window as I sped toward her house. She went to the door, only to watch in horror as I flew by without stopping. The throttle lever had caught itself between two of my jacket buttons, and there I went, completely out of control, beating and flailing at my chest in an attempt to free my jacket before I crashed into a tree. It was very exciting, in a Pee Wee Herman sort of way—"Dean's Great Adventure." But it isn't something I want to have happen very often. So, the jacket has to have a zipper with no buttoned, snapped, or Velcro-fastened storm-flap.

Finally there is my own personal aesthetic. I don't want to settle for a jacket that "works" as far as function is concerned but simply doesn't appeal to me. Oh, I know there's an awful lot that's more important in this world than what someone with MS is going to wear this winter. This isn't even my greatest personal difficulty with *having* MS. But I reflect on how thoughtlessly I used to choose what I'd wear before MS. Aesthetics could dominate my thinking because function was a given. I could wear any coat designed. Now I have to work to balance function and appearance. Well, another two or three coats are due to arrive this week. I've already made many compromises in adjusting to life with MS. I'd like to think that somewhere out there is a jacket that will see me through fall and winter warmly, safely, conveniently, and in style, here on Cripple Creek.

The Turkey

MY SISTER received a free frozen turkey for Thanksgiving from her local grocer. Because she had plans to dine out on the holiday, she thought she'd offer it to charity. She called several organizations, but apparently, everyone in the USA had received a free turkey for Thanksgiving and had attempted to do the same. Apparently, all receivers of charity had also received free turkeys and wanted no more of them. If I understood her correctly, people below the poverty-line have been running, screaming, at the sight of a median-income person approaching them with a turkey. It's a wonder that the turkey industry makes any money!

I, too, had purchased enough at my food store to qualify for a free frozen turkey. I got mine a week before the holiday and, having no oven of my own, planned to bring it to my friend Sue for her to cook in her convection oven. And then I planned to give her half of it—my version of charity. She agreed to that. I have the weakness and poor balance associated with multiple sclerosis, and I staggered as I lugged this 18-pound frozen turkey (the smallest they had) from the store to my car while store personnel smiled encouragingly and wished me a happy Thanksgiving. Then I lugged it from my car to Sue's and went home to take a nap. She put it in the fridge to thaw. During the three days it took to thaw, Sue realized that she didn't have room in her convection oven for a bird this size. She also has a regular gas oven but hadn't used it in several years. (It had become, essentially, a bread-box, warm and dry, where she keeps crackers; in winter it sometimes houses mice, in spring, snakes.) So our mutual friend, Barton, came and got the turkey, cooked it for us, took a share, and returned the rest to Sue. Sue took a share and handed off the remainder to me. I took mine home and was sick of turkey within a few meals. I ended up giving much of it to the dogs and to some wild little fur-beings outside. So, you could say that most of my turkey fed those less fortunate than myself, although, given how weary we all became of eating turkey, I believe we were all equally unfortunate.

I have come to believe that turkey is a dish requiring some very long-range planning. Between the time it takes to thaw, the time it takes to slow-roast, and the seemingly interminable time it takes to consume, one can start to imagine seeing one's children through toddlerhood and schooling, until they are grown, educated, and married. And even at that there will probably still be a drumstick lurking malevolently in the back of the fridge.

After the Fall

(WRITTEN IN OCTOBER, 2001)

THIS LATE AUTUMN, although I want to continue spinning amusing tales of life with MS, I feel totally uninspired. Since the events of 9/11, many people have felt a deep sorrow. I am among them.

On the day of the service in the National Cathedral, I went to my own place of worship. It's a small country church and no one else was there. I sat in the sanctuary and cried. I can't even imagine the terror felt by the people in the targeted buildings or on the airplanes. I can't imagine the desperation and, later, grief felt by those losing loved ones even as they spoke together on cellular phones.

I also wept for the lost innocence of Americans as a people. Our national character has been formed, to some extent, by our security—our distance from hostile powers and our essentially egalitarian society. We'd been described by other nations as bumptious, gregarious, (too) open, and self-centered. We were like children, assuming everyone loved us, and not understanding when they did not; we were egocentric and greedy, not in an evil way, but in the innocent way of children. As a nation, we will never be that carefree again. I am not saying that this is good or bad. I don't know how to value it. But it is a loss. And while we are being encouraged to toughen up and dig in for a protracted "war on terrorism," I expect we may also need to grieve our lost innocence just as any child traumatized by assault would need to do.

Afterwards, I went to the local Wal-Mart to buy some much-needed household items. While I recognized the solemnity of the day, stores were open and I wanted to combine trips. I try to do as many things as possible when I'm out and about, to more efficiently utilize the limited energy that MS has left me. It was a national Day of Mourning, but my critters needed to be fed and other, more personal matters needed seeing to. Our Wal-Mart has television monitors hanging from the ceiling throughout the store. Usually the programming consists of advertisements for store products. On this day, however, the monitors were showing the service in the cathedral. All over the store were teary clumps of customers and employees gazing up at the monitors with rapt attention. Other employees were at their registers or were stocking shelves in a desultory way. And, here and there, a lone customer sadly trundled a cart in an aisle. Trundling my own cart, I found the dog food I needed and then went on to my "more personal matters." The aisle containing bathroom tissue is at least 30 feet long and 11 feet high I can't begin to count the brands and qualities of the paper sold there. It comes in double rolls, triple rolls, two-ply and single-ply, quilted, scented, unscented, with aloe, in 8, 12, 16, and 24-packs. We live in a country that offers us umpteen-gazillion choices of toilet paper!

And I thought about the people in Afghanistan, who have nothing left after years of strife and violence. I don't imagine they are concerned over the quality of bathroom tissue. I don't even know if they can take the availability of such a thing for granted. I thought about what had happened in New York City and Washington D.C.—all those people, suddenly gone forever, who had gotten up that morning and, in confident anticipation of an ordinary day, had used the product of their choice. I stood in the aisle at Wal-Mart still grieving our nation's lost innocence and, paralyzed by the sheer number of offerings, was unable to decide which to purchase. And as I stood there, someone in the National Cathedral began singing "The Lord's Prayer." This pretty completely undid me. I hastily chose a package without looking to see what brand it was, how many rolls were in it, or what sort of rolls they were. I felt ridiculous, but I also felt completely, typically, even *quintessentially* American. I paid for my purchases at a register manned by an employee seemingly distracted by sorrow, and came home to Cripple Creek.

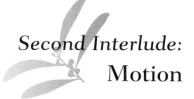

Second Interlude:
Motion

MS HAS CHANGED both the way I move and the way I *think* about moving. Most of us with relapsing/remitting MS aren't visibly disabled, particularly if we are holding still. Despite "looking so well" (which many of us are often told), we experience a variety of abnormal sensations and varying degrees of bodily dysfunction. In my own case, I have times when I can be spastic, limp as a wet noodle with fatigue, dizzy with vertigo trying to walk straight ahead but falling to one side or the other, or staggering as if drunk. Sometimes I am all of these at once. Numb fingers can cause me to drop things, miss picking them up altogether, or feel that I have something in my hand when I do not.

I've experimented with a variety of aids and techniques to help maintain at least some of my physical competence, and I've made many changes in my daily life to accommodate the physically crippling aspects of my MS.

These five essays describe some of my experiences in the areas movement and the activities of daily life with multiple sclerosis.

She Flies Through the Air

DUE TO THEIR SIMPLE vocabularies and lack of sophisti-
cated grammar, young children often hear things incorrectly—song
lyrics and so forth. Certain words and sentence structures are not
yet in their repertoires, so they substitute whatever makes sense to
them, often with amusing results. For instance, I have a friend who,
before she learned to read, sang a hymn called "Gladly the Cross
I'd Bear" with great enthusiasm as "Glad Lee, the Cross-eyed Bear."
A young boy I know, conditioned by catchy advertising jingles,
thought the Kenny Rogers and Dolly Parton duet, "Islands in the
Stream," was "Island Industries." I grew up watching a woman on
TV who possessed the absolute coolest name possible. Yes, on
weekends at my grandparents, we tuned in *not* to "The Dinah
Shore Show" but to the "Dinosaur Show." What five-year-old could
not adore a woman named *Dinosaur*? The daughter of a nurse, I
also believed that the daring young man on the flying trapeze was
incapacitated by grave illness and, thus, I sang, *"He flies through the
air with the greatest disease..."* Little did I know that, with a change
of pronoun, I was describing my own future trajectory.

Incapacitated by the MS symptoms of vertigo, poor balance,
and spasticity, I have, on occasion, flown through the air myself.
Some of these flights follow, ironically, on the heels of an obser-
ver's positive comment. Not long ago I saw my internist. The last
time she'd seen me, over a year before, I was using two canes.
On *this* day, however, I was walking unassisted. I trailed her down
the carpeted hall to her office. "Gee!" she exclaimed over her
shoulder, "you're walking really well!"

63

"I sure am!" I agreed. My reply was followed by a muffled thump as I measured my length on the carpet behind her.

Someone suggested that using a cane might have saved me a spill. This is not necessarily the case. One day, I left an appointment with my therapist calling a cheery "Good-bye!" as I closed her office door behind me and stepped into the (thankfully, as it turns out) empty waiting room. I was using a cane that day, but my spastic foot swung into the cane, and I lost my balance. As I began my descent to the parquet floor I reached toward one of six bamboo and wicker waiting-room chairs. Too light to take my weight, it joined me in falling with a loud clattering noise. Another of the chairs, caught by my cane, came along as well. My momentum carried me and these two chairs across the slick wood of the floor and into the chairs on the other side of the room. I can't believe this went unheard by my therapist (*"There's that client, acting-out her neediness again!"* I imagined her wearily sighing). But I'm grateful she didn't emerge from her office. It gave me time to untangle myself, put the chairs and their cushions back in order, and make my exit in face-saving privacy.

There was a time earlier in my life with MS when I'd stumble and catch myself. If out in public, I'd look around in embarrassment to see if anyone had noticed my clumsy move. As my reflexes have become less reliable, I no longer simply stumble nor have I any hope of not being observed. No one in the hotel lobby where I fell during one Christmas season could have avoided noticing me. I tripped and, trying to regain my balance, began a staggering lurch across the lobby. In desperation, I reached for the hotel's Christmas tree as I lumbered past it. With my keys and purse contents spewing and my walking appliance flailing, my eventual fall had only a tad more subtlety (and made only a tad less noise) than the overly decorated tree would have, had *it* fallen. I just missed my grab or an empirical comparison might have been possible.

An old chestnut of philosophy asks us, "What sound does a tree make falling in a forest if no one is there to hear it?" If the tree is anything like me, the sound it makes is, *"Oh, shit! I'm falling."* Unlike me, the tree gets but one opportunity to say this in its lifetime. I, with myriad opportunities, usually finish my sentence with *"again."* I *feel* like a tree when I fall these days. I've seen a slow-motion tape of trees coming down and in my imagination I look just like that—the straight trunk going from perpendicular to parallel in its relation to the ground, the bounce as it hits. They say that during an accident, one's perception of time slows. When I'm on the way down, I seem to have time to notice the surface I'm about to hit. Is it hard? Will it hurt? Will it tear or stain my clothes? I have time to review my daily "To Do" list and decide which tasks I'll probably have to forego as a result of this fall. If I had my cellular phone, I'd probably have time to call someone and say *"Oh shit! I'm falling, again."*

There are ways to fall safely. One of the first things one learns in martial arts classes is how to do this so as not to hurt oneself. Indeed, one must fall, ready to rise again and immediately resume combat. Football and soccer players become adept as well. As a girl riding horses, I was taught to fall without danger. Before my MS became symptomatic, I could tuck and roll as I fell—going with the fall and, for the most part, avoiding bodily harm.

With reactions compromised by the disease, however, I can no longer rely on those skills. These days, I risk serious injury when falling, the more so as I age. So, even if I am *able* to walk, there are now times when discretion dictates I use a wheelchair or scooter, perhaps when I'm on unfamiliar terrain where falling is more likely and sitting makes more sense. Sometimes I use a chair because I'm dressed well enough that I'd prefer not to chance ruining my outfit or denting my dignity. I don't mind taking a tumble in easily replaced sweats and jeans made for grimy pursuits, but the potential damage is more expensive in a twin set and pearls. In addition, the contrast between a graceful appearance and a graceless fall is distressingly incongruent to me.

Nevertheless, as long as I am on foot at all, I recognize that my probability of falling is greater than average. On any given day, you may find me stumbling and tumbling onto the wood-chipped path to the barn, tripping and flopping into the creek, or overbalancing on my shovel and subsiding into the garden loam. Often, it's taken significant injury, lost teeth, or broken bones, to convince many people with MS that walking is more of a liability than it's worth. The ground is pretty forgiving here on Cripple Creek, though, with no cement or concrete surfaces. I've grown accustomed to mud and grass stains on my farm clothes and, at this point, I'm pretty much able to relax as I fly through the air with the greatest disease. This I do without a net, reveling in the gasps of amazement from friends and family members. So, I'm not sitting down for good—not just yet.

Into the Closet

AT ONE TIME I lived a simple, low-tech life here on Cripple Creek. As my MS worsened, I added a cane. It was wooden and had a curved top. As far as canes went, I thought it was the best one could do, state-of-the-art and all that. Gradually, I acquired a *selection* of canes; business-casual, dress, sporty. Go on, laugh, but it's true. I have a nice black cane with a dark wooden t-grip handle. Because it's adjustable, I can choose to wear heels or not. It's the sort of thing to carry on a dinner date. For the great outdoors, there's an aluminum trekking pole, also adjustable, with a built-in antishock setting. It has an intricate, airbrushed design of Victorian curlicues and flowers in bright red on a black lacquered background. It looks cool and people stop me to ask where they can get one. I also have a shorter, blue and silver trekking stick with a cork t-grip handle. More sedate than the stafflike pole, it's used for everyday outings. For use when hanging out with the granola-and-sandals crowd, I have a handmade cane, the handle carved into the shape of a fish. I even have a cane with an attachment at the bottom with retractable sharpened prongs for use on ice! Lately, I've been eyeing some lovely flowered aluminum canes with hardwood handles. They're a bit more feminine than the trekking poles and would coordinate beautifully with summer outfits.

There was a time when disabled and chronically diseased people were kept hidden from the rest of the world, locked in institutions and asylums, living in basements and attics, their existences alluded to in whispers. Such people were the objects of pity and horror in Gothic literature. They were construed as demonic (as in some of Flannery O'Connor's stories) or as diamonds in the rough (read *The Secret Garden*, by Frances Hodgson Burnett), depending on the author's need. Franklin Roosevelt, one of the first visibly disabled persons in public life, gave fireside chats from a wheelchair. In that circumstance, radio, a nonvisual medium, kept him sequestered from public view. Although activism and political correctness have resulted in a greater degree of public accessibility, allowing more of us to be out and about, the physically challenged have not truly become an accepted part of mainstream consciousness.

That seems slowly to be changing. I've seen disabled people pictured using the products in mail-order catalogs such as L.L. Bean, represented by mannequins in department stores, and as characters in TV serials ("*West Wing*" comes immediately to mind). There are upscale clothing and equipment catalogs exclusively *for* the disabled (check out *Rolli Moden*). But the most *seductive* change is in the number of catalogs offering relatively inexpensive gadgets and aids to promote health, fitness, and independence. One doesn't necessarily see disabled folks pictured *using* these things, but the implication is there. I imagine this plethora of choices is due to the deep pockets of aging baby-boomers, but we with MS can certainly reap the benefit. Some of these items look like so much fun one might almost wish to be disabled, just to have the excuse to need them. Since I *do* need them, I had to have a try despite the inner voice which told me things, especially *advertised* things, are often not what they claim to be. When it comes to gadgets, my *joie de vivre* tends to overwhelm my *caveat emptor*.

In one catalog, I saw an adjustable-tension pedal-exerciser that sits on the floor. The ad copy told me that, from the comfort of my chair, I could pedal my way to fitness *"Now there is no excuse!"* it said. The accompanying picture showed an elderly woman reading a book in an easy chair, her feet on the pedals of this machine. Having been told I had no excuse to avoid doing so, I bought one. I followed the instructions for setting the tension, placed it before my chair, picked up a book, and sat to pedal. The contraption slid away from my chair and, since my feet were strapped to the pedals, I quickly joined it on the floor. I tried putting a rubber mat beneath it. This time the mat and the exerciser slid away *together,* although I was savvy enough to avoid following. I managed to eliminate the sliding by placing bricks on one end of the machine. However, I found that the force of pedaling lifted the unweighted end off the floor and sent the bricks themselves sliding away. They were immediately joined by the rubber mat and the machine. No matter what I tried, I could not use the exerciser with the ease that the catalog promised. I've come to believe that the older woman pictured in the catalog was using this piece of equipment as a foot-rest. It was a still photograph, after all. I didn't actually *see* her pedaling. Discouraged, I put the pedal-exerciser in the closet.

I bought a gripper/reacher that was advertised to allow one to pick up anything from a dime to a can of soup. There was a picture of its little rubber tips pointed toward a dime on the floor. There was a picture of a man, his arm outstretched, using the gripper to hold a can of soup. The man was apparently the current Mr. Universe. It never occurred to me that a can of soup held at the end of a gripper was going to weigh so much! Had I paid close attention to local squirrels, as thin branches bent beneath them, I might have foreseen what would happen next. My arm dipped. I had trouble holding the gripper closed. The can of soup slipped, fell to the floor, and rolled under the table. *"I could have done that without this gripper,"* I sighed. As for the dime or any other small object, I soon realized that to pick them up off the floor, you first need to be able to *see* them. I put the soup cans on a lower shelf, became accustomed to crawling on the floor wearing reading glasses, and sent the gripper to the closet.

I bought something that you clip onto the shaft of your cane. A flat extension projects to the side of the cane's shaft with a rubber button top and bottom. You can slide the clip up and down the length of the cane. It allows you to balance your cane vertically on the edges of counters instead of leaning it precariously or trying to hold it while making purchases or writing checks. The clip can be slid under a table's edge, creating a tension that holds the cane vertically beside you as you eat. The pictures showed the cane balanced on a counter's edge and standing jauntily at table beside a seated restaurant customer.

The cane with its clip and I went to dinner with my friend Barton. "Is that new?" she asked when she saw the clip. I told her it was and demonstrated, as I took my seat, how easily it slid beneath the table's edge to hold my cane at the ready. "Great!" she said, jiggling the table as she sat down. The cane, thus released from its tension, fell beneath the table. I replaced it. It fell again when the waitress bumped the table. It fell when she put the dishes down. It fell when I brushed it with my leg. It fell when a heavy-footed diner passed by shaking the floor. When the meal was over,

I strolled up to the counter to pay the bill. Using the clip, I perched the cane on the edge of the counter. "That's interesting," said the counter-person eyeing my clip, "What does it do?" The cane rocked once on its fulcrum and clattered to the floor. "Nothing," I cheerfully replied. Back home, the clip joined the pedal-exerciser and the gripper you-know-where.

These three things have since been joined by several other disappointingly useless aids to independence, among them the *lifting cushion* that is placed on a chair and offers a boost when one wishes to stand up quickly and fling oneself headlong into the next room; the glasses that, refracting at a 90-degree angle, allow one to read as if seated while lying on one's back nauseated from disorientation; and a folding cane that, taken out of its sheath and shaken, snaps into usefulness once and each time thereafter flops dejectedly at the end of one's arm, refusing to assemble itself.

These failures have dissuaded me from continuing to buy and try some of the more arcane things advertised, yet I find that canes and their accessories still fascinate. Just today, while glancing through a catalog I caught myself staring appraisingly at a new cane that purports to easily grasp a table or armchair by means of a *"hidden built-in mechanism."* It features an ABS handle (one hopes this does *not* mean *antilock braking system*) and promises to eliminate the "embarrassment of fallen canes." We've already got commercials for shampoos that prevent the embarrassment of baldness and pills that prevent the embarrassment of *decreased vitality* (as it's coyly described).

As the current generation continues to demand youthful independence in the face of encroaching age-related disability, I'm anticipating a television commercial in which disabled restaurant-goers, each using one of these wonderful canes, smirk, snicker, and nudge one another while a diner not-so-equipped stares in shame at her cane, which has fallen noisily to the floor. In another TV ad the camera might pan, from behind, a row of fellows sitting on bar stools each with his cane at attention beside him, Tammy Wynette's *"Stand By Your Man"* wailing on the soundtrack. I'm glad we cripples are coming out of the closet. *My* closet, at any rate, continues to make room for the storage of items purchased in seeming defiance of the adage that a fool and, in this case, *her* money are soon parted.

If the Shoe Fits

HAVING WRITTEN of my attempts to find a suitable winter jacket, I now offer this series of vignettes concerning shoes.

When I was first diagnosed with MS, I refused to believe the doctor. I had no reason to believe him because, as often happens early in the course of the disease, in a few weeks, I was back to normal, doing all the things I'd been doing before my attack. And, as I had all my life, I wore whatever I thought looked good on my feet.

After several years, I found myself dragging my left foot when I walked more than a mile or so. Of course, this was not a sign of my MS returning. It was a sign that I wasn't wearing the proper footgear. I bought myself a better (i.e., more expensive), more supportive pair of hiking boots.

The new boots didn't help. When other symptoms began to appear, I saw a different neurologist. He confirmed the initial diagnosis of bygone years. He said my foot problem was caused by spasticity. He explained that when one's leg muscles tense, they actually extend and make the leg longer. If this happens when one is walking, in a spastic moment, one leg suddenly becomes longer than the other and the long one "catches" on the ground. He suggested I buy a pair of high-top tennies to help prevent my foot from extending in spasticity. Well, I *still* wasn't very accepting of the diagnosis, but I do like buying shoes. So, I bought a couple of pairs (hey, they were cheap) of Converse Chuck Taylor All-Stars.

But my leg continued to try to extend, and now it was "fighting" against the sneaker. This was actually very painful. And, instead of helping me look cool the way these sneakers do on younger folks, I found myself heading toward the little-old-lady-in-tennis-shoes category. What's more, you can't wear sneakers everywhere you go when you're a middle-aged woman. So, since I like shopping for shoes, I continued my quest with credit card in hand.

I decided I'd be able to walk just fine if only I had enough room in the shoe for my spastic toes to flex and stretch. I decided the spasticity was being caused not by MS but by shoes that were *too tight* (ain't denial grand?). So, I bought men's shoes a size larger than I would have needed even if I'd regularly worn men's shoes. I wear a women's 7½ and I bought a men's 8. Go figure! I had room. *By golly*, I could have held a group therapy session in each shoe (and I probably should have). Well, they stayed on, provided I wore enough socks, but I really couldn't walk in them. I could shuffle. My foot no longer caught on the ground because my foot was now unable to *leave* the ground. I felt (and looked) like one of those inflatable weighted clowns that bounce upright again when punched. Only, of course, when I fell over, I didn't bounce upright again. I just lay there. However, I knew now that the reason I couldn't walk was that my shoes were *too big*.

I next entered what I will call "The Sandal Period." In the correct size, sandals gave my toes plenty of room to flex and stretch. Sandals with a back strap stayed on my feet (don't even talk to me about slides, mules, or clogs). Sandals come in all sizes and styles. There are sandals for hiking, water sports, dress up, casual hanging out, working on the farm—for every occasion except winter (although there are special socks and waterproof sock-covers for people who insist on wearing sandals in winter). Believe me, I know this because I now own these things. But sandals, especially with their winter adaptations, were not very appealing aesthetically.

That meant I had to buy winter shoes, right? For winter, I bought sheepskin boots made specifically to be worn without socks. Leather on the outside, they are fully lined with deep wool pile that takes the place of a sock. There's room for spastic toes to flex, there's wooly warmth in winter and, as with the sandals, they look age-appropriate. But, *darn it all*, neither the sandals nor the boots were helping me *walk* any better! So I hadn't yet found the solution. Knowing that there's no problem that can't be solved provided one approaches it clearly and with open-minded honesty, I thought long and hard before realizing that *moccasins* could be the answer. Did I mention that I enjoy buying shoes? After all, moccasins go back a long way as footgear. They've been worn by people who historically did an awful *lot* of walking.

I could continue this saga with several more attempts on my part to solve the "I can't walk well, it must be my shoes" problem. I could discuss special walking shoes and how I reasoned (at one point) that, since they are called "walking shoes," I ought to be able to *walk* in them. I could write about special European-designed toe-boxes on shoes made for the cobbled streets of European cities, and Scandinavian "comfort footwear" (apparently there is an entire industry in Scandinavia devoted to the comfort of American feet). There's even an expensive collection of shoes made by a company called "Mephisto." Remembering that Mephisto is another name for Satan, I told myself the devil was making me buy the shoes. And now, I can only say that there isn't a shoe to be found that is going to improve my walking. I know this because I have an example of every shoe ever made. I could (and may) open a shoe museum.

The drug baclofen, prescribed to relieve spasticity, has definitely improved my walking. Using a cane or staff has also improved my walking by giving me better balance and minimizing side-to-side lurching on my more symptomatic days. At some point in the future, a leg brace may help, although it isn't necessary at this time. With these approaches, I'm finally getting real. I have learned, through much trial-by-shopping, that MS isn't caused by ill-fitting shoes, nor will shoes of any kind make MS go away. Call me the "Imelda Marcos" of Cripple Creek!

Cleanliness Is Next to Impossible

WHEN I WAS A CHILD, my mother had a woman in to clean the house once a week. In my middle-class family, this was considered a sign of our having some sort of elevated status with regard to material well-being. It also meant that, for the most part, I was not trained to care for a home. For many years after I left the nest, through college and early working-life, I continued not to care for my various dwellings, nor had I anyone in to clean for me. The resulting conditions in which I lived are best left to the imagination. (You may entertain sticky linoleum, environmental microniches with their own flora and fauna in bathrooms, and dust-bunnies the size of actual rabbits.) Of course, I was a student and then a wage slave, and most of the places I could afford were half-way to derelict with no help from me.

As my earning power improved, so did my choice of housing and, eventually, I came to build a house at Cripple Creek. While that house was being constructed, I lived in a rented farmhouse. Middle age, vanity, and an interest in meditation combined at that point with the result that, in a 180-degree turn, I started taking an interest in cleaning my living space. I began to respond to the objects and surfaces with which I dwelt. I saw dusting and polishing as a way to express gratitude for what I had. A fresh and tidy home seemed more welcoming to friends, I now believed. I'd heard of someone called *Martha Stewart* and became convinced she held the keys to my destiny. It was a good thing I'd come to enjoy cleaning because, what with all the decorative projects producing an endless parade of knick-knacks, I soon had lots to clean, shine, polish, dust, and arrange.

I continued in this vein as I moved into my new house. As is often the case with me, I went to extremes. I developed expertise, of a sort, in all the products available for efficient home-care and was able to bore people at gatherings with, for example, my knowledge of the merits of different laundry aids. People who visited were amazed (and probably a bit intimidated) by the state of my rooms. They commented on how clean and beautifully decorated the house was, and I modestly (but nowhere near modestly enough) accepted their accolades. When I went to visit others, they apologized for the dust and grime they were sure I would observe. In, truth, though, I really didn't care what other folks did with their homes. I barely noticed the state of my friends' dwellings. I was fanatic only about that of my own.

MS symptoms creep up slowly sometimes, particularly after a long remission. In the years following my move to Cripple Creek, I noticed that I was too tired to do certain jobs I'd always been able to do before. I eliminated the decorative crafts projects first. Gradually the collection of objects was thinned. I didn't have the energy to care for all that nonsense anymore. I'd get tired carrying the vacuum cleaner up and down the stairs. I began to divide the cleaning chores between two days rather than getting it done in one, as had been my habit. I can't recall the task with certainty, but I remember hearing myself say (I *do* talk to myself when cleaning alone) *"Oh, that doesn't matter so much. No one will notice,"* the first time I decided to remove something completely from the list of chores. I also began to remove furniture from the house. What did I really need besides a table, two chairs, a bed, a desk, and an easy chair? Because I lived alone at the time, I had complete freedom to make these decisions. Finding bed making too exhausting, I decided not to change the linens every week. I stopped washing the floor. I stopped dusting areas that required a step stool to reach. Plagued by dizziness and poor balance, I staggered from room to room, lurching into walls and grabbing at the remaining furniture, a rag and a bottle of lemon oil in my hand. I had numerous area rugs and had formerly envisioned myself sitting contentedly on them playing with my dogs. Now, although playing on the floor was still an option, getting up again was not. It had become too difficult for me to shake or vacuum these rugs and their bunching and sliding were, to the dogs' surprised delight, landing me on the floor more often than I wished. I folded the rugs away.

One day, I looked into the bathtub and the thought of getting on my knees to scrub it clean practically reduced me to tears.

A famed book of spiritual practice promises that as we are created from dust, we will eventually return to dust. It was happening much sooner than I'd expected. I began to pay someone to clean for me but, as you know if you've ever been skilled at a task, no one else does it quite the way (i.e., *as well as*) you do. Along with many of the other MS-related changes I'd accepted, I now had to come to terms with this.

I was aided in my adjustment by being too tired to care much about house-cleaning one way or the other. There were a few clumps of dog hair under the bed? So what? The sink was a little grimy, and the house-cleaner wasn't due for another week? Well, at least the plumbing was working. I found that my denial, formerly employed toward *not noticing* MS, could be redirected toward *not noticing* uncompleted household tasks. Not knowing when or to what degree I would become disabled, nor how long I'd remain so, I had to completely reselect my values to allow me to be engaged, as much as possible, in what truly mattered to me. Housekeeping didn't make the cut. If I could be active for only a few hours each day, I decided to spend my few hours standing in the woods. I paid a different kind of attention to those around me, and noticed that people who valued themselves, people I adored and respected, lived in contentment in less-than-pristine houses. It seemed that, perhaps, if one felt clean and tidy on the *inside,* one's perception of the outside would pretty much take care of itself.

I haven't returned to my student days in my attitude toward home hygiene. There are no attack-trained dust-bunnies waiting to grab the ankles of those who visit, and mycologists will find nothing of interest growing in my bathroom. But, I *am* more relaxed and forgiving about what needs to be done to run a household and, although once again in remission, I have continued with my revised, less fanatic standards of good stewardship. I'm thankful for what I've learned about myself in the process, and I remain open to the lessons of my teacher, MS.

You Wear What You Eat

A WHILE AGO, there was a commercial on television that showed a woman whose hind parts consisted of two round Danish pastries and a man who couldn't get through the turnstile in the subway because he had a chocolate-covered doughnut where his abdomen should have been. The commercial advised healthy nutrition in the form of a particular product the advertiser wished you to buy. The poor people so depicted had become what they ate for breakfast, and no one needed to guess what that was.

No one need guess what I eat, either, but for a different reason. Whether I'm carrying a mug of tea from the counter to the table, twirling a fork filled with sauce-soaked pasta, or stabbing a celery stick into veggie dip at a buffet table, I'm bound to end up with reminders of my meals on my clothing. Were I a writer of Proust's caliber, I might conjure an entire novel based on a food stain from a meal long past and forgotten, but now rediscovered on an old woolen sweater.

Spasticity is my constant companion, and it may become less controlled (even with medication) in a social situation when I am excited or stressed. A simple act like walking while carrying a bowl of soup can easily result in embarrassment for me and smothered mirth for my guests. Over the years, while entertaining at home, I have been mopped clean by many delightful people who then agreed to order dinner in. Some of these people have become good friends. I have also been mopped by solicitous, clucking waitresses in restaurants. Being female, and with respect for the bounds of social propriety, I do not allow *waiters* to mop me. I have also spent an extraordinary amount of time mopping *myself*.

One can try to dress for the type of food one anticipates eating (reds and oranges for tomato-based Italian dishes, pale shades for light-colored dips and seafood, browns and taupe shades for curries and Chinese cuisine). Tweeds and plaids are good. They were invented for concealing warriors and hunters in the wilderness of ancient Britain. Surely, they can now conceal whatever falls upon one from the table? When it comes to knits, it is a good idea to buy sweaters with "marled" yarns, yarns of different but complementary colors twisted together. I became aware of this one night when I'd spilled a caramel latte on a tan-and-natural marled-yarn sweater I was wearing. The spilled beverage didn't show after it had soaked in well. Black is usually a safe color to wear. It lends an air of sophistication—and I need all the help I can get if I'm going to accessorize with the appetizer. Black slims one's appearance (which plaid assuredly does *not*) and, once you wash the food off, the wet spot left is less revealing on a black garment.

When dining with others, if conversation lags, one can offer oneself as a subject for wager. People can place bets as to when the first stain will occur, how many stains will be accrued during the meal, or of what food the first stain will consist. This can be a delightful way of enlivening a meal. It relaxes people when you poke fun at yourself, so that when you *do* spill food, your companions need not risk apoplexy by trying to suppress their guffaws.

I have three adult bibs. They are reversible, with one solid side and one printed side. They are designed to look like vests and have nice details in the form of buttons and pockets. They fasten with Velcro behind the neck. One of mine is a black sateen-finished cotton for more formal occasions. The other two are a banker gray (less formal) and a sage green with a Hawaiian print on the reverse (downright casual). I hardly ever wear them because they are *bibs*, for gosh sake! But I *think* about wearing them, and I wish I *had* worn them each time I bid goodbye to one more ruined garment.

I have learned a great deal about stain removers. It's always best to treat the stain as soon as it happens, if possible. To that end, I have my favorite stain remover in every room of the house, and I carry some in my purse.

As I write this I am reminded that it's just about time for a snack with my neighbor. I can anticipate spilled iced coffee and melted chocolate crumbs ground into whatever I wear, so I believe I'll wear the brown trousers! *Bon appetit*, from Cripple Creek!

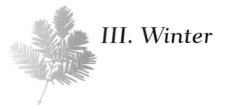

III. Winter

ALTHOUGH NOT MY FAVORITE time of year, winter on Cripple Creek has its charms. I enjoy decorating for the holidays, and I enjoy holing up indoors with good reading material while the dogs snooze by the fire. I continue to spend time outside when the weather permits, and I watch the winter birds at the suet feeder and appreciate the more subtle shades coloring the woods and fields.

We don't get much snow here, but when we do my scooter, with its four-wheel-drive, remains in use. I'm able to walk in snow, although I find it to be very tiring. The cold weather can contribute to an increase in spasticity and, with reduced activity outdoors, I find it important to do some regular stretching and to get as much exercise as I can handle to avoid losing the muscle-tone I'll need for next spring's farm chores.

Each of the next essays was written during the winter months.

Demolition Shopping

I AM OFTEN STUNNED by the ignorance and obliviousness I find in the design of stores and public buildings. Some businesses have notions of "accessible" that make me shake my head in wonder.

How about automated storefront doors that have those handy metal buttons you can slap? Easy, right? After you slap the button mounted on the wall of the building beside the door, you have to race over to the door itself because it doesn't open wide enough for you to wait where you are. It often has a threshold lip that will hang up your wheelchair. Some of the cheapest models have a timed open/shut cycle (like an elevator) and there you sit, trying to rock your chair over the lip only to be pinioned between the closing doors. Some malls near me have doors that open in or out! Got a manual chair? You hit the button and BOOM! You fly backward with fractured knees. (I'm surprised more of us aren't millionaires, given the lawsuits we might initiate.)

One financial institution not far from Cripple Creek decided to install a ramp so that customers in wheelchairs or scooters could get to its door, which sits above a short stone staircase. The ramp is cement with railings and three (count 'em) *three* switchbacks. The space allowed for turns in those switchbacks is too narrow for many scooters. Additionally the switchbacks are *left on a slant* rather than being level. So, if you are in a manual chair and need rest on what feels like a three-mile ramp to the bank? Well, for you mythology buffs, let's just say that I refer to the place as The First National Bank of Sisyphus, and I deposit my money elsewhere.

"Ah, stop complaining and go to the drive-through window!" you might advise, *"Save your legs and arms some energy."* I *do* use the drive-through window whenever I'm in the mood for ab crunches, because the bank's deposit drawer is so far below the window of my wheelchair-accessible van that I have to lean *waayyy* over to get anything in or out.

Some curb cuts have a half-inch drop-off at the bottom. It's quite a jolt going down one of these in a manual chair, and next to impossible to come up one. A friend tried to push me from street to sidewalk on such a cut and, unaware of the bump, almost dumped me on my face.

When shopping in larger stores, I have often used one of the scooters so considerately provided by the business. Controls for scooters are not standardized, as they are for other forms of trans-portation. Some scooters have thumb-operated toggles below the handlebars. Others have handlebars that you twist one way for *forward,* the other way for *reverse.* Some have push-levers mounted *on* the handlebars. So, when you go to a store, until you are familiar with their machines, you never know what sort of controls you'll be using. Thus, just as one gets physical exercise negotiating the obstacles resulting from ignorant barrier-free design, one gets intellectual exercise learning all the different ways of driving a scooter.

I have had many zany adventures shopping from a scooter in major discount department stores. I commend these stores for nice wide aisles, but they have a propensity for stacking displays down the centers of those nice wide aisles, thus creating two nar-row aisles on either side of the display with no regard for accessibility. At the end of each of these now non-negotiable aisles, they put "end-cap" displays that make it impossible to see anyone entering or leaving an aisle. The products themselves are stacked so high that my choices are usually limited to a few shelves below able-bodied eye-level. This is not where the more popular brands are kept. So I cruise carefully through the store selecting things that aren't quite what I want but are what I can reach, trying to avoid running anyone over as I enter or leave an aisle and keeping in mind which driving configuration my scooter has. Sometimes, however, things go awry.

I was in such a store one day looking for socks. Women's socks are in the Women's Lingerie Department, which has teensy crowded aisles with lots of flimsy, lace and elastic-laden things flapping about loosely. I got stuck. One handlebar of my scooter became entangled in a display. This kept it locked in drive-mode and, as I moved helplessly forward, I pulled an entire carousel of brassieres down. They draped themselves over me and the scooter. I was appalled. Thus festooned, grinning with embarrassment and muttering apologies, I explained to the salespeople who came over to glare at me that I'd only wanted some socks. (*"What do cripples want with socks, anyway?"* my paranoid mind interpreted their looks.) They watched impatiently as I tried to untangle myself and back up. The Women's Lingerie Department is next to the Jewelry and Accessory Department and, reversing in the too-small space available to the scooter, I ran into a display of sunglasses. Although nothing broke, it made quite a sound as it went over. I'd now attracted an even larger number of annoyed salespeople, so I decided to forget about socks and get out as quickly as I could.

I headed for the nearest exit. This happened to be in the Lawn and Garden Department, where the doors opened *outward* rather than sliding apart. I could have gone back into the main store area and found a sliding door. But that would have meant passing the scene of destruction I'd created. So, instead, I politely asked a salesperson to hold the door for me. This she grudgingly agreed to do. The threshold had a lip and I knew I'd have to gun the scooter to get it over on the first try. I sure didn't want the experience of an already sullen salesperson becoming even more sullen as I sat there trying to ram the scooter over the threshold. So I gave it all it had. The scooter responded with energy and flew right over that threshold. As it did, the back fender brushed against a display of glass-topped patio tables stacked on end in huge cardboard boxes way too close to the door for a scooter to pass by safely. Each box took its own sweet time sliding away from the others and crashing with a thump to the floor. Each box pushed the one before it a little further until the first box reached a display of barbeque utensils and knocked it over. Talk about noise!

The sounds of mayhem faded behind me as I scooted to my van. I was ashamed and sorry, but I was also irked with the store for making my shopping experience so difficult. Maybe someday, businesses will come to terms with the true meanings of "barrier-free" and "accessible." Meanwhile, with the holiday season soon upon us, let's all head out and do our best to hasten that day.

Making a List

THE WINTER SEASON'S holidays can be stressful. Most of the references I've come across on the subject talk of depression for the lonely, the strain of dysfunctional family gatherings, and onerous obligations. But stress doesn't attach itself only to unpleasant circumstances. Stress can result from *any* change in routine—even a darned good one! While holidays can be stressful for anyone, we with MS do well to take *particular* care of our health during this time. We need to be vigilant in our awareness because, often, a lot is required of us during the holidays. MS is a disease that can leave us with less to give just when more is asked.

One way I handle the demands of the holiday season is to prioritize, limiting or eliminating tasks and activities I deem unimportant. For example, I go to the closet to get the Christmas lights out only to realize the closet is incredibly cluttered with the ghosts of Christmas past. I find broken strings of garland, pieces of Styrofoam that used to be ornaments, an old photo album filled with pictures from bygone holiday parties, and (let's admit we all have a few of these) hideous holiday knick-knacks received as gifts and never to be displayed. Instead of using my energy to clean and sort through these useless unwanted things, I spend three hours engrossed in the photo album trying to remember the names of most of the people in the pictures. No, that's not what I do. That would not be a suitable use of my limited energy. I hastily withdraw the necessary lights and slam the door on the disorganization. I know the mess can wait until after Christmas. I am saving myself for those things I really wish or need to do.

I try to delegate if possible, allowing friends and family members to help so that I can be fully present rather than too fatigued to enjoy the festivities. Most of my family members are dogs, but even dogs can make a contribution. While mine often help me accessorize my party outfits with shed hair, they're best at cleaning up after meals. They also enjoy cleaning up before and during meals. An unattended holiday buffet table is their delight. Guests wandering about with full plates of food are also a great favorite.

During the holiday season, along with my lists of gifts to buy and things to do, I bear in mind a symptom checklist to use as a guide. My old familiar symptoms wax and wane as I undertake too much and then, realizing the problem, cut back to where I am more comfortable. Although I have a pretty full, low-level complement of MS symptoms, a few seem to worsen more quickly under stress. In my case, they are spasticity in walking, poor balance, dizziness, and numbness in my hands and feet. I particularly monitor these during the holidays.

I notice an increase in spasticity when I'm excited about some approaching event for which I have the primary responsibility, such as company coming. I'm usually pretty physically active while getting ready to entertain, cleaning, shopping, and cooking. But I do those activities at other times, too, without a problem. I associate my increased trouble walking during the holiday season with *anticipatory pleasure* or, perhaps, *anxiety* as to whether the affair I planned will come off. You'd think after all these years I'd have realized that things will *never* go as planned or, rather, that I'd learn to plan for the way things *do go*. Often I become less spastic once the event is unfolding. Instead, I'm putting my effort into resurrecting the toppled buffet table, breaking up the dogs' arguments over fallen food, and finding a place that delivers party trays on very short notice. I put up with the spasticity while getting ready to entertain since I know it will soon be obliterated in whirling party chaos.

Balance problems are most likely to increase when I venture into unfamiliar territory, going out to a concert or restaurant or visiting in someone's home. Spasticity isn't a problem at those times, but I *do* have trouble keeping my footing. I tend to move more tentatively in unfamiliar space, as does anyone. My feet are generally somewhat numb and my vision is compromised by optic neuritis, and these factors probably combine with cautious steps to throw my balance off. At parties in other people's homes, I try to find some place to sit instead of mingling. A person with MS balance problems carrying a full plate of food and a glass of beverage can give a new and unpleasant slant to the word *mingling*. Although I stay seated and let the party come to me, sooner or later I need the facilities. These are usually upstairs and, as I often say, I'm not truly at ease in someone's home until I have fallen down their staircase. With familiarity, my balance improves (although wise men say you can never fall down the same staircase twice). Again, I don't worry about the worsening balance difficulties during holidays because I know they are not permanent. They are simply a response to situational stress and, although normally I don't absolutely need one these days, I wish I didn't almost always forget to take a cane with me into such situations.

The increase in the other symptoms I listed seems to be an

after-effect of stress. I am likely to suffer from dizziness as well as decreased sensation in my fingers and feet on the day after the event. In fact, I use those symptoms as a measure of how good a time I've had. The more fun, the more dizziness and numbness the day after. This is my own little MS hangover, and the best cure for it is rest. If I haven't remembered to take it easy following a stressful holiday undertaking those symptoms are my *heads-up*. Ignoring them, I risk falling head-down and injuring myself, as happened one December 26. I was dizzy, and my extremities were numb. I was paying no attention though, partying fool that I was. Returning home from one last event, I sat on a stool to pull my boots off, unbalanced myself, and fell backward off the stool. That tumble resulted in a mild concussion. Now I am more *attentive* to my need for down-time after parties. I don't have to worry about these symptoms as long as I recognize their message and respond appropriately. I know they will subside within a few days.

I've had MS for many years. That's a lot of time to process the comings and goings of symptoms. I've learned which ones are fairly constant, which ones are periodic with no apparent reference to life's vicissitudes, and which ones seem directly related to stress in their intensity. I've learned to distinguish a mild increase in old symptoms from a relapse or attack. I'm not always *totally* sure or clear on these distinctions. But most of the time I'm certain enough.

So, check yourself out, if you don't already do so. See how well your body's working and what's "iffy" as the next holiday season approaches. Make a list and know what to look for. Decide which of your symptoms are parts of your "early-warning system" and which are the dues you pay for having a good time. Plan for time out when you need some. Many of us can keep going if we get some solid rest time between activities. Share your knowledge with family and friends so that they can respond helpfully when you notice a stress-related symptom increasing. Looking for a great holiday gift? Caring well for yourself is the gift that keeps on giving.

On Turning Fifty

I'VE JUST HAD MY 50TH BIRTHDAY. When I was diagnosed with MS back in 1984, I was told I'd likely be confined to a wheelchair within 25 years. That would have put me at about 58, an age so distant then, that I couldn't imagine reaching it. The neurologist made this pronouncement in a cheerful tone, as if 25 more years of walking ought be considered a bargain. I believe the words "It's not so bad" preceded his statement. But those early symptoms subsided and didn't return for several years of blithe denial.

When my MS reasserted itself more intensely in the early 1990s, I went to a neurologist for the first time since 1984. I'd thumbed my nose at the original diagnosis, but now I was scared. Maybe I really was on my way to wheelchair confinement. Despite the fact that I was having a lot of trouble walking, the neurologist I saw this time said that my case was a very *mild* one and that there was no reason for me ever to need a wheelchair. I was relieved, because I was much closer to my 50s than I'd been in 1984, and I really wasn't ready to sit down more or less permanently. As it turned out, however, both of these doctors were wrong—or both were right, depending on one's point of view. I *do* need a wheelchair now for anything involving long distance, and I can still walk in the house and for short distances outside. Thanks to the injectable pharmaceutical I've chosen, I may be able to walk farther, and for more years, than anyone could have predicted in 1984.

In fact, when it snowed one day, just a few light, powdery inches

96

here on Cripple Creek, I was able to shovel a path to ride my scooter to my neighbor's house. Now *there's* a typical MS picture: A passerby sees me out shoveling. *"What are you doing?"* they ask, *"I thought you had MS!"* *"Well, yes, I do have MS,"* I reply. *"I'm shoveling this path for my scooter so I won't have to walk."* They look at me as if I'm crazy. But the truth is, I have just enough coordination and energy to do this little bit of shoveling, and then I'll need that scooter to get to and from my neighbor's as I often do. If I didn't shovel the path, I wouldn't be able to get there at all. And, although many people I know were crabbing about having to shovel snow, I was smiling because I still *could* shovel this little bit.

So, for me, MS hasn't been the disaster it was predicted to be when I was first diagnosed. Although I can no longer deny the impact of MS on my life, I can look forward to more years of walking *short* distances or shoveling a *little* snow. In thinking about both my fears of disaster and my subsequent denial, an old family birthday story comes to mind. It contains elements of both denial and disaster. Long ago, my mother insisted to me, from her perspective as an older and wiser adult, that one day I'd look back on these events and laugh:

My mother had grown up in a close family, in an urban environment, and had been a very popular child. She and my father moved to the suburbs shortly after their marriage and, when I came along, she naturally wanted me to have friends and be popular, too. I was not a popular little girl, though. Physical clumsiness and social awkwardness kept me on the outskirts of childhood cliques. My mother felt that this situation could be changed for the better and to that end, she invited several little girls from my class to go out to lunch and then to a movie as a party for me on my tenth birthday. In those days, people were generally polite in accepting invitations and the little girls duly arrived, somewhat ungraciously, on the appointed day. Although not terribly pleased with the context (my birthday), the girls seemed willing enough to be entertained. My birthday falls close on the heels of the winter holidays and, as I look back, I imagine that, in addition to their dislike of me, they were probably jaded from various celebrations and school vacation treats.

My mother, heavily girded in denial, greeted these taffeta- and crinoline-clad little girls with great good cheer, loaded us all into my family's ancient sea-green Studebaker, and we headed off. The little girls chose not to address me but, instead, giggled among themselves. I thought they were probably making jokes about me. My mother heard only the sound of happy voices and completely overlooked the content.

Things quickly went from relatively uncomfortable to extremely so. Someone requested music. The knob fell off the radio when my mother reached to turn it on. The little girls rolled their eyes. There would be no music. We wouldn't have been able to listen anyway because the car began making a horrible noise and belching black smoke. My mother merrily insisted there was nothing wrong with it. The little girls rolled their eyes again. When a dashboard alarm light came on, Mother decided to go to a gas station we'd passed a block back. She explained that we would miss lunch at the restaurant, but we'd go to the movie after the car was fixed, and could eat popcorn and candy there..."*Wouldn't that be more fun than lunch, anyway?*" The little girls rolled their eyes some more. Mother's attitude was that going to a gas station in a malfunctioning car was high adventure, and we should all get in the spirit. She pulled into an alley to turn the car around and, in backing out of the alley, knocked the mirror off the driver's side door. She joked about this as if she'd done it intentionally to amuse us. She pulled the groaning, shrieking car, trailing its kamikaze tail of filthy smoke, into the gas station and opened the door to get out. The door fell off the car and landed like an up-ended turtle on the tarmac. My mother, who by now had *really* pushed the denial-envelope as far as she possibly could, gave up and burst into gales of semi-hysterical laughter. The little girls' eyes seemed to spin around completely, as their heads did 180s on their little necks, *à la* Linda Blair in *"The Exorcist."* Their mothers were called to come pick them up.

My recent fiftieth birthday was an important one, the beginning of a new decade for me and a new millennium for time-keeping humankind. Friends asked me to suggest an activity that would most please me. I replied that I should like to go to dinner and a movie in a well maintained and mechanically sound vehicle with someone who cares for me. I did so, and on the way home, I told this story. As has often been the case, Mother was right.

Observations On the Search
for Companionship

THE OBSERVATIONS that follow are, I believe, as applicable to those looking for a romantic attachment as to those who are, as I was, simply looking for a close, enduring companionship.

Someone once wrote to me and described the attraction of a person he recently met with this quote from Thomas Merton: "He had a simplicity of spirit preserved by the will to be true." Reading that letter made me wonder just what it is we require of ourselves and each other in order to be found acceptable, even loveable, in all our relationships.

For any couple, MS is a difficult disease to come to terms with. Of course, there are couples that do *not* come through a diagnosis of MS together, but if the partnership is a good enough one, and there has been time before the diagnosis to build trust and caring, a couple may negotiate the difficulty successfully. There seem to be at least *some* adequate written resources for people who live in families, for caregiving companions, and for couples concerned about "intimacy" and the effects of MS. MS used to be a disease most frequently diagnosed in a person's mid-thirties, and the majority of people diagnosed were, perhaps, assumed to be in whatever relationship they wished at that point.

MS is diagnosed in younger people these days, and the single person with MS, alone for whatever reason, faces a different set of circumstances. With few written resources, this person must choose whether, when, and how to offer MS along with whatever other qualities are brought to a potential relationship.

I once lived alone with MS. For many of those years, I worked on coming to terms with the disease and rebuilding my life to accommodate it. When I thought about relationships, I reminded myself that life on Cripple Creek is sort of isolating—good for the personal work I was doing, but not so great for meeting new friends. However, one winter's day, I realized that what I really wanted, more than anything, was to live in companionship. I wanted someone to cook meals with and share the events of the day. I wished to share my life with someone to whom prayer and meditation were as important as they'd become to me. Being very clear that I was *not* looking for romance, I placed online a few carefully written "personal profiles," as they are sanitarily called.

Recall the adage: "You can't judge a book by its cover, for it's what's *inside* that counts." When beginning any sort of relationship online, unless pictures are immediately exchanged, you really do offer the *inside* that you hope will count before you offer the *cover* by which you're hoping not to be judged. Even when pictures have been exchanged, unless you are photographed using an assistive device, people are apt not to see that you have MS.

Each of us has probably heard many times, "But you look so *good!*" If you have MS, this compliment has particular poignancy when planning to meet in person someone you've discovered online. You must decide beforehand whether or not to mention MS. I tried the up-front approach once or twice and never heard from those correspondents again. So, the next few times, imagining bits of personal information as pebbles dropped into the clear pool of a new friendship, I chose not to heave the boulder of MS. One of my real-time acquaintance sarcastically asked, "Well, when are you going to mention it—when they visit and see the *stair-lift?*" I had to find a middle ground. I developed an "out-of-the-closet-with-MS" paragraph and introduced it gradually into my written exchanges. This seemed to work well, offering each correspondent a chance to freak out, recover, and then ask questions, at a comfortable pace.

I also put myself in the way of meeting people in non-virtual venues. Isolated though I am, I do get asked to parties and other gatherings. MS is a different matter when meeting someone at a party or in another live context. I was advised by one person to wait until I felt confident enough to bring up the subject of MS. But if your MS is visible, you may not have that luxury. If you use a walking appliance, there it is. If spasticity causes you to stumble and fling your plate of food in the air, there you are, stumbling and flinging food.

When these things occur, you may be asked what's wrong. This provides an opportunity to mention MS. Then it becomes a question of *how* to present it. That may depend on how far in accepting the disease you have come, whether you're having a good day or a bad day, on the situation in which you have just *met* this potential friend or love of your life (are you wiping flung fondue off the person's chest?), and a multitude of other factors (such as how loosened your tongue has become due to overconsumption of party beverages).

The reactions of those with whom I spent time ran the gamut from instant rejection (eyes wandering, temperature dropping, dry-cleaning bill forthcoming—you know the signs) through varying degrees of acceptance. Among those who chose to continue with me, some wanted to know right off the bat whether they risked becoming mired in nursing duties or otherwise responsible for me should my condition deteriorate significantly during the course of our friendship. They were afraid, and that is how they chose to verbalize their fears. Some wanted to cure me, or wanted me to cure myself and could not believe I was doing all I could to take care of this disease. They were also afraid and used criticism as a defense against their fears. Some people trivialized MS. Trivializing is another way of handling fear. Beginning any kind of relationship, romantic or not, is scary enough for two people. They put themselves out there for judgment while, at the same time, each tries to judge the suitability of the other. What a balancing act! To some extent with MS, one is always contending with one's own fears about the disease. Mention MS to potential intimates, and you must deal with their fears as well.

It's been an ongoing struggle and adventure for me to come to terms with who I am as a result of MS. I'd come to feel fairly content with myself in isolation. But at the thought of opening myself up to another person, I found myself considering the ways that MS had foreclosed opportunities for handling companionable pastimes conventionally. I wondered what I could offer to replace, for instance, outdoor sports activities, staying up late at night to talk, traveling on the spur of the moment without making arrangements for a wheelchair, or running together across a sandy beach and diving into the sea. How could I invite someone to play? And what of accomplishments and talents? Often, "What do you do?" is the opening gambit for a possible future connection. I happened no longer to be making a conventionally recognized contribution to society, nor was I engaged in a high-powered career and earning a salary. What to say? For some, there may also be physical concerns, such as a body studded with site-reactions from injectable therapies, or the presence of incontinence pads in the bathroom.

MS forces us to take stock of what really matters, to cease doing some things we believed were important, and to make peace with letting go in order to conserve our limited strength and energy. The advantage of having done this myself is that it allowed me to do the same, to some extent, with others as well. As a result, I found myself more accepting of another person's ways, and much less judgmental than in pre-MS days.

I've found it important and helpful to describe myself primarily on the basis of my strengths in the here-and-now, and to talk about the valuable work I've done in coming to terms with MS. I spoke of my volunteer work on behalf of others with MS, and of my faith and its place in my life. When I had to talk about limitations, I stated them matter-of-factly. I was not completely at ease when having to acknowledge these, but I took my cue from an old dog-trainer's advice: *Begin as you mean to go on.* I decided it was better to put my limitations on the table. Reserving them risked my becoming symptomatic at an inconvenient time, to another's dismay.

As stated earlier, when I began my search for a companion I wasn't looking for conventional *"til-death-do-us-partnership."* I hoped for a close, enduring, and spiritual friendship that would both accept and transcend my disability. Many disabled people desire such a friend in their lives. For some, this comes as part of a traditional marriage. For others, there are less conventional romantic attachments. There are those who find hired companionship works well. There are also many other ways for people to connect and share. My openness to this fact improved my chance of finding what I sought. Along the way, I met several very interesting people both online and off, I had fun, and I eventually met someone with whom I now share my life. Thus, the adventure continues and Cripple Creek flows on.

Third Interlude:
Community

So, I NO LONGER LIVE ALONE. But, in truth, I never did—not completely. There have been family members, both chosen and God-given, to enrich my life. I have continually enjoyed friendships that matter to me. And the companionship of dogs has been important to me as well. The person with whom I share my present life is a crowning gift, one that I cherish.

With visible disabilities due to MS, I often find myself interacting with complete strangers in public as they stop to offer assistance or ask me about my assistive appliances. This sort of interaction can create community where none might exist otherwise. It affords me the opportunity to educate and to deepen awareness of the personhood of crippled folks in those not so afflicted.

In these next essays, I focus on MS at it affects my relationships with others, directly or not, for better or worse.

Turn About

AMONG THE DOGS here at Cripple Creek is an old West Highland white terrier named Griffin. As Westies go, she's not much to look at, having been rescued from a puppy mill and having no great lineage. She's been my companion for many years, and I love her dearly. I got her as a pet originally, but having grown up around dogs, I decided to offer her obedience training during her formative months. She did well in her basic class, although, being a terrier and stubborn as all get out, she handled some of the exercises "creatively." After that eight-week course, we went home and pretty much forgot about formal training. I was employed full-time in those days, and my situation allowed Griffin to accompany me to work.

When she was four years old, I decided to return for a more advanced obedience class with an eye toward entering Griffin in trials. I thought it might be fun to be out and about among dog-people. Griffin had proven herself a public-spirited girl, well-socialized by this time, and she enjoyed entertaining people. After some struggles together over how the formal obedience-trial exercises ought to be performed, Griffin and I became quite a team. Although I really didn't enjoy standing in the ring before a judge at a trial (the very words "judge" and "trial" give me the willies), Griffin completely gave herself to the experience, loved to show off, and eventually we earned two American Kennel Club titles.

Then my MS got worse. It had been in remission for so long that I had decided I didn't have it. But several symptoms gradually began to intrude. My gait became more and more uneven.

Eventually, I really couldn't walk far at all. I became weak. I fell down a lot. There were two attacks of optic neuritis. No longer able to trust my body in the show ring, I retired myself and Griffin from further competition.

One day, I took a walk in the woods with several people and our dogs, six-year-old Griffin among them. The trail was a loop of a mile or so. I thought I could handle that using my cane. The friends I was with got ahead of me as I began to walk more and more slowly. Then my feet stopped lifting, and all I could do was shuffle them forward, tripping over small obstacles on the path. Finally, even shuffling was too much and I stood still in the woods, alone.

Griffin had been rollicking ahead with the rest of the dog pack. But she was always well attuned to me, and she circled back to find me. It was very peaceful standing there leaning on my cane. I didn't dare sit for fear I'd never get up again. Griffin knew something wasn't right. She encouraged me to walk, to chase her in that way dogs have of running toward you and then away in short bursts. Nothing doing, though. I just stood there. So she took off. And she was soon out of sight. I assumed she'd gone back to play with the dogs but, as my friends later told me, here is what she did:

Griffin ran to the other humans and stopped a few feet behind them and whined. When they turned to look at her she was standing in a very still and alert position and she barked at them. She dashed away, stopped, turned, and barked again. She did this repeatedly, until one of them (no doubt remembering the old "Lassie" TV show), got the hint. Griffin then led my friends back to where I stood and they helped me out of the woods and back to the car.

After that, I began training Griffin as an assistance dog. She learned to go get a neighbor if I fell or got "stuck" outside in the woods and fields. She was tested and certified by an agency that trains assistance dogs in a three-hour, grueling examination of her skill and steadiness in all sorts of public situations. With her certification, she was able to go everywhere with me—movies, dinner—you name it, she went. And several more years passed.

Who knows why things happen as they do? My MS stopped progressing. I began to show improvement. I no longer needed an assistance dog. And for her part, Griffin began to age. She developed arthritis, and jumping into the car became hard for her. So there we'd be at the grocery store, the crippled lady and her assistance dog. We'd finish shopping and walk to the car. I'd then have to lift her into the car. "Ha-ha!" someone would chortle (usually me), "Who's the cripple?"

Griffin is thirteen as of this writing. She's stiff, getting cataracts, going deaf, and showing signs of senility. No one meeting her now would understand my adoration of her, for her glory-days have passed. She still loves to play outdoors, to ride in the car, and to be fussed over with praise and food-rewards. Her insistence on those last considerations can make her seem spoiled, unless you know the context in which they came to be part of how we share together, she and I. These days I suppose you could describe me as her assistance-human. I look out for her, guide her when she becomes disoriented, lift her where she can't jump, see that she gets her share of treats, and make sure she isn't forgotten among the more robust members of the Cripple Creek pack.

As I sat down to write this essay, Griffin lay down behind my chair with a cookie to chew. I was worried that the chair's castors would hurt her if I moved, and I asked her to shift away. She didn't hear me, so I leaned down and slid her further from the chair. She looked offended as if to say, "*Well!* You could have just *asked* me to move!"

"I *did* ask you," I replied, "but you didn't *hear* me. Who's the cripple?"

"Goes around, comes around!" said Griffin. I agreed and passed her another cookie.

Doctor, Doctor

WHEN ONE IS DIAGNOSED with an incurable, progressively crippling disease, well—it's hard to digest that. The first thing *I* wanted to know when told I had MS was whether it could be cured. The answer was, as it is now, *"No."*

"Well," I asked, "if you can't cure it, what can you do to prevent it?"

In the early 1980s the answer was, *"Nothing."* No-one wants to hear that a doctor can't really do much for them. And I don't suppose many doctors want to view themselves as relatively useless, either. It upsets the natural order of things in which one gets sick, goes to a doctor for treatment, and is cured. That's the American way, and we've almost all been taught to expect it.

Although I've heard some with MS speak admiringly of their neurologists, I listen to many more describing their doctors as brusque, uncaring, never returning calls, not having time to answer questions, unwilling to try new or "alternative" treatments, dismissive, and even disbelieving of their patients. To mitigate against this situation, we are advised to educate ourselves, make lists of questions ahead of a doctor's appointment, shop around for a compatible neurologist, and become assertive in requiring our doctors to take us seriously and to treat us with respect.

The doctor–patient relationship can be a loaded one, into which the patient may bring the unresolved longings for safety and protection from harm that every person carries within. Doctors may transfer similar buried longings of their own onto their patients. Onto the smoldering tinder created by that dynamic is thrown the log of MS, where there's no protection or safety to be had. In the resulting emotional conflagration, it is no wonder people spend a lot of time seriously trashing their neurologists.

I feel very sorry for my neurologist. In my imagination, he became a doctor in order to be of service to sick or injured people. Doctors must derive *some* career satisfaction when they are able to cure or fix people. And my neurologist, *in my case*, can't do that. I really like my neurologist. He's not an MS specialist, but he's very well-informed and keeps up to date on recent research. He also thinks for himself and doesn't jump on the latest treatment bandwagon. He allows me to think for myself as well. It's a good fit, and I consider myself fortunate.

I first saw this doctor several years after my diagnosis, on the advice of my internist. She saw that I was becoming symptomatic and referred me to a neurologist. I was conflicted about the reality of MS beginning to assert itself in my life. I didn't want to—*I was not going to*—be helpless. I marched through the door of his office, armed with all the information about MS that my reading eyes could absorb, sure of my own opinions and, leading with my chin, obviously unwilling to be influenced. I imagine this perceptive man took one look at me and thought, *"Hoo boy! Here is a woman who does NOT respond well to male authority figures. I'd better lay low."* And in that, he was absolutely right. He's continued to lay low over the years. For instance, when he sent me for an MRI, the technicians were running late, and I had another appointment to get to that day. In addition, I didn't particularly want to be a person who *needed* an MRI. Given this state of internal affairs, I somewhat arrogantly refused to finish the series. He accepted that and made do with what they'd managed to get in the time I was willing to spend. On another occasion during the first year of seeing me, he tried to suggest one of the injectable therapies. Not wanting to admit my fears both of needles and of *needing* needles, I responded with an angry list of trumped-up "scientific" reasons why I didn't *"need no stinkin' injectable therapies."* He didn't push.

Two years later, when I decided I ought to be on one of them and asked his opinion he said, quietly, "If it was me, I'd have been on one two years ago."

By then, I'd become gracious enough to forbear saying, "Well, it *isn't* you, is it?!"

He's a practical guy. He advised a pair of high-top tennis shoes as a less expensive way to control drop-foot than a brace. He's recommended naps for fatigue and a cup of coffee to offset the initial dopiness I felt when trying a new drug for spasticity. All of these were simple solutions, relatively inexpensive, and easily available.

He's a city-boy, though. And I am most definitely neither. I called to ask him whether I ought to get a vaccination against Lyme disease. "Nah," he replied, "Just stay on the sidewalk and you won't get ticks."

"Um, doctor," I said, "I live in the woods, for pity's sake! We don't have sidewalks out here." Another time, I had to argue with him for a prescription for a scooter. He didn't want to seem to encourage my becoming dependent on such a thing until I explained that I live on a farm where there are chores to be done at some distance from my house. "If I walk to the chore-site carrying whatever tools

I need to do the job, I'll be too tired to do the job by the time I get there," I told him. I got the scooter. In neither case did he mean to respond inappropriately—he simply had no clue.

There are those with MS who prefer seeing their doctors often to discuss the waxing and waning of their symptoms and to review the treatment options available, even if there is nothing more to be done. Seeing the doctor gives them the sense that an effort is being made. Unfortunately, *because* there's nothing to be done, their doctors may seem disinterested—even irritated by such patients' importuning. Others have many more complications than I do, or more rapidly progressing MS, and really *need* medications tweaked and therapies attempted. For such people, a neurologist's care can result in a more comfortable adjustment to life with MS.

But I like my neurologist for leaving me alone. He will certainly give me whatever help he can, provided I ask. And although I don't ask for much, I try to keep informed so that I know what to ask *for*. The last time I saw him, we decided not to have a second MRI because, as he put it, "If it shows disease activity, we're going to keep you on your injections, and if it shows no disease activity we're still going to keep you on your injections. So it doesn't really matter." My neurologist and I go our separate ways, willing that the best be done on my behalf and, at the same time, gracefully accepting some helplessness in the face of an incurable, progressive disease.

The Uncertainty Principle

MS DOESN'T ALWAYS display itself, especially in the early stages of the relapsing-remitting form. Even when the disease has progressed, MS may not be visible if one is keeping still or sitting down. We are often told how *normal* we look. Sometimes this is said in a tone of reassurance (*Don't worry about your progressive, incurable neurologic disease—you're still attractive*). At other times, it's said somewhat resentfully (*What right have you to claim to be disabled when you look so healthy?*). It's as if, in order to be acceptably disabled, one must make the contribution of being physically unappealing or must pay by wearing some sign—the scarlet C of Crippledom. Conversely, if one is not going to do that, one may be suspected of not being so very disabled after all.

People who come to visit me, whether or not they know me well, find it difficult to understand why I have a stair-lift, a manual wheelchair, a scooter, and a walking staff. If I'm having a good day and am not using any of those appliances, they find it hard to accept that I might need them on another day. They can't comprehend why I have such a variety of options. Further, they often seem not to trust my *own* perception of my degree of disability on any given day.

Mistrust and suspicion seem to be common experiences between those of us who have MS and those with whom we interact. One might expect this from total strangers, but the list of those who mistrust us often includes medical personnel, friends, and family. Having MS, we have learned to live with untrustworthy "wiring," often unsure what our capabilities will be from one time to the next. And we live *inside* our bodies! It must be even more difficult for someone who hasn't the experience of a body with MS to really know what it's like. Of course, we try to imagine how it is for our loved ones, and they do the same for us. But that doesn't make being mistrusted any easier to tolerate.

Illness is a liability in a society with a frontier mentality. I can't speak for other nations, but it seems that in the USA, with its overt history of doughty settlers and immigrants escaping poverty elsewhere, we have a pioneer orientation that gets summed up as "every man for himself." This is not a particularly compassionate national philosophy. As a nation, we are not given to helping citizen-victims of *social* misfortune in a nonjudgmental, unconditional way. We don't even quite believe in *victims of social misfortune*, but prefer to see all people as captains of their own destinies and to judge those whose ships are sinking as "bad" captains. Thus, one who can't "paddle his own canoe" can expect to be left behind with little or no succor from society. Many of you who've applied for disability insurance are well aware of this, especially if you've faced an appeals board.

The political becomes personal in our own homes and among our acquaintances. Our loved ones don't want us to fall by the wayside. They want us to keep up, to stay the course. So, they have an investment in *not* accepting our disabled status. For some there may also be an element of "damaged goods" involved (there is no TV show called "*Who Wants to Marry a Cripple?*"). It's easier to mistrust the one with MS who says "I can't do that today" than it is to deal with the sense of having chosen badly. No one wants *their* friend, husband, or wife to be the one left behind while the wagon train moves on. And, since society values competition over compassion (except at worship services), it stands to reason that a loved one might feel burdened by the need to develop a compassionate response to a disabled partner or friend. It's often easier to mistrust this person's need for compassion—or, anyway, what's perceived as "need." In truth, most of those with MS whom I know are not gratuitously needy at all. Most of my acquaintances in the MS community are doing whatever they can, sometimes way more than is healthy, to preserve their independence.

But still the mistrust is there. It's there in our friends and family members, and it's there inside ourselves as well. In the end, I keep coming back to the idea of uncertainty. When you're close to someone who has MS, that closeness may challenge your ideas of what you really do control. With MS one learns experientially what people pay gurus and Zen masters for—to ride with the tide, to live in the moment. Most people are not compelled by circumstances to learn this lesson, and wouldn't choose MS to *have* to learn it. But when you *have* MS, the quality of your life may *depend* on learning it.

We with MS are no better than others. We get discouraged, frustrated, angry, and defensive. But many of us do learn to *let go*. Heck, many of us can't even count on getting out of bed from one day to the next and putting our pants on one leg at a time. The uncertainty we experience, and the mistrust it generates, might be among the gifts of MS—a challenge to each of us to help those who are close to us to become more open to, and accepting of, uncertainty in their own lives as well as in ours.

And tomorrow, whether or not I can get out of bed and put my pants on one leg at a time, I and my loved ones will continue learning the lessons of MS here on Cripple Creek.

Walk This Way

THE SONG "Walk Like an Egyptian," written in 1985 and recorded by the Bangles, gives an amused nod to an old Three Stooges movie "The Three Stooges Meet the Mummy." In the film, Larry, Moe and Curly meet an Egyptian mummy in a tomb where they're looking for hidden treasure. The mummy offers to help them in their search, inviting them to follow him with the words *"Walk this way."* He proceeds them down the hall of the tomb, walking stiffly sideways as do the people depicted in Egyptian paintings. As is the case with them, the Stooges take his command literally and fall in behind him, imitating his distinctive walk.

Shortly after I was diagnosed with MS in the mid-1980s, I was contacted by a social worker from the hospital where the diagnosis took place. She called to recommend I attend an MS support group that met in a small town west of Cripple Creek. She was concerned by what the diagnosing physician had reported as my *ho-hum* attitude, and she wanted to make sure I got all the help I needed to adjust to the bad news I'd received.

Being a fairly agreeable gal, usually up for a new adventure, I agreed to go check it out and, on the appointed day, drove to the address she'd given me. Upon entering the meeting room, I was greeted by the sight of several people in wheelchairs. I'd never seen a powerchair before and, to my anxious and uneducated eye, these looked less like modes of transportation than like advanced life-support systems. Some of the people were strapped or braced into their chairs. Others, not in chairs, had crutches on their arms and braces on their feet. I was welcomed by the group's leader. We sat around a large table, and they commenced to talk. I was so unnerved by the degree of disability among those surrounding me that I took in very little of what was said. Adding to my incomprehension, several people had speech difficulties that made them hard to understand. In fear and loathing, I left the meeting as soon as was reasonable, vowing inwardly never to return. I told friends on Cripple Creek (none of whom has MS) that *those* people were much worse off than I, that they spent too much time complaining about their problems, and that I didn't need a group such as theirs because I wasn't disabled. The thing that frightened me most was that they had been smiling and had seemed to take pleasure in their community. *"How could they?"* I wondered. In retrospect, I'm aware of the selfishness of my response. I believed, blindly, that they had nothing to offer me, and I was unable to consider what I might have offered them.

After recovering from my first attack, I spent ten years in ignorant and blissful denial. Gradually, my symptoms began to reassert themselves. As they became more frequent, they wrought changes on both my abilities and my body-image. I became disabled enough to require a cane on good days and a wheelchair or scooter much of the time. I did not feel good about myself and, beginning to come to terms with what seemed inevitable, I recognized a need for support. On my own this time, I contacted the National MS Society and was directed to a group that met in a large city south of Cripple Creek.

On the appointed day I drove my ramp-van to the address I'd been given and entered the meeting room, moving slowly with two canes. I was greeted by the sight of several people much younger than myself, all in apparent good health with no visible disabilities. There were no powerchairs, no canes (other than mine), and no braces. All of these folks were in early-stage relapsing/remitting MS and all were using one of the new injectable therapies (which I, at the time, was not). We sat in a circle and commenced to talk, but I was so unnerved by the lack of disability surrounding me that I took in very little of what was said. Adding to my incomprehension were the pharmaceutical and medical terms sprinkled liberally throughout the conversation— words like *interferon*, *site-reaction*, and *subcutaneous*. When I trotted out my ersatz spiritual acceptance of the gradual erosion of my abilities due to MS, they looked at me with fear and loathing. *"How can you be enjoying so compromised a life?"* they asked in wonder, *"How can you not be on one of the new therapies?"* I left the meeting as soon as was reasonable, vowing inwardly never to return. I told my friends that *those* people were much better off than I, that they spent too much time crowing about how well they were doing, and that I didn't fit into a group such as theirs because I was older and wiser about disability while they were still in denial. In retrospect, I'm aware of the selfishness of my response. I never considered that, in return for whatever they had to offer me, my visibly disabled presence might have been a gift to them.

Several more years have passed, during which I've become intensely involved with others who suffer MS via an online chat that I co-host at *www.msworld.org*. Perhaps the fact of physical privacy in an online venue makes the difference, or it may simply be that time and hard work on defects of character has improved me. At any rate, I now number many with MS among my virtual acquaintances, and I'm comfortable with the widely varying degrees of disability among those afflicted. I both get and give support in my work online and some of those with whom I work at MSWorld have become my friends. I'd met but a few people with MS in person, however, and those few not in a group situation.

I've also begun using one of the available injectable therapies and am convinced I owe much of my relative well-being to having done so. I've entered a time of remission and, although I sometimes use a cane, I'm often able to walk with no aids at all. With medication to relieve spasticity, my gait is sometimes almost normal. But I still have many days when I walk as one neurologically impaired— particularly when excited by an event or when under the stress of unfamiliar surroundings.

At the invitation of a colleague, I recently agreed to speak at a meeting for women with MS hosted by a local chapter of the National MS Society. I'd never done much public speaking, but I'm still an adventurous gal and, thus, on the appointed day I drove to the designated site and met the colleague who'd invited me to join her in speaking.

Some twenty-five attendees were present, all seated as the program began. For the most part, they were middle-aged, just as I am. Some of them had braces on their feet. Most had canes, some with forearm cuffs. Two of the women were in wheelchairs. They all listened to our presentation and participated eagerly in the discussion that followed. In that discussion, we spoke of how MS had changed our lives, and of how each of us had been forced to rethink her direction when the disease made its entrance. We spoke of the gifts of MS—how the disease had offered each of us opportunities to make behavioral changes that she might not otherwise have made. I listened with deep appreciation to the conversation as it swirled around me and felt wonderfully energized by this experience. What I had to offer was enthusiastically received, and I was given a great deal in return.

Then the group broke for refreshments. One by one, or in small groups of two and three, the women made their way to the buffet table. Until then, we'd been using words to express our shared experience of MS. But now I saw that each of them walked, as I do, with a stiff, slowly tentative gait. Each of them moved, as I do, as if her balance might fail her at any moment. I felt no fear or loathing viewing this display of disability, only joy at finding a final manifestation of what we had in common. I stood with my cane to join them and, unable to find the coffee pot, asked one of the participants where it might be. *"Walk this way,"* she invited. With a huge grin, this happy stooge did exactly as she asked.

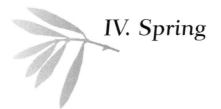

IV. Spring

No matter what is happening in my life with MS, spring on Cripple Creek never fails to lift my spirits. I'm entertained by the burgeoning population of wild beings, both those returning from winter sojourns in the south and those newly born to permanent residents. I've come to know and appreciate the variety of wild plants that grow here and look forward each spring to the season of their blooming.

I often experience a flare-up of my MS during the first warm days, until my internal thermostat adjusts to the change in ambient temperature. But once I've adjusted, and until the heat of summer begins in earnest, I look forward to some of the most symptom-free days of the year in weather not too cold, not too hot...just right!

These last four essays are from four different, but equally rewarding, spring seasons.

Shifting Gears on Shifting Sands

SPRING IS COMING to Cripple Creek. Geese are on the move. Song birds are singing different songs from those sung in winter. Donkeys and sheep are braying and baaing to their new babies on the farm across the valley. As the equinox approaches, the angle of light changes. It's an old saying that nothing is certain *except* change.

Just about the time I make a definitive statement about my MS, I can be sure that whatever I've attempted to nail down will change. I tell someone my legs are too spastic to walk. The next day they see me out strolling along with my cane. Often we with MS are felt to be either malingerers, outright liars, or totally deluded. Sometimes, we are accused of using the excuse of disease to manipulate others. It's hard to hold onto one's inner truth because it really *can* change, sometimes from one hour to the next. I might be too tired to do the dishes and an hour later *not* be too tired to go out to the movies. Is that the disease at work? Is it within my control?

It's a blow to find you can't rely on your body as you once did. It's a different sort of blow to find that you can't even rely on your difficulties staying the same from one day to the next. We're so used to being in control, making plans, and following through, keeping to a schedule. The workings of our entire society (at least in the USA) are based on such behaviors. My golly, we even have schedules and systems for handling grief! The stages are outlined for us and defined. Although it's not suggested that we progress through these uniformly, I've found myself observing, of someone, *"Gee, she's been in denial a long time! Shouldn't she be moving into anger soon?"*

So, perhaps more immediately than other people, those of us with MS have to learn to handle sudden change. Having MS can seem like driving through a desert with ever-shifting sands. We try to make our lives work despite changing symptoms and cycles of exacerbation and remission. Our bodies stagger uncertainly and our disease does the same. What was there yesterday is gone today. What is gone today may be back tomorrow. We count on the understanding of loved ones, on support groups, and on caring medical professionals (when we can find them). Some of us develop strong spiritual practices to which we can bring our distress and uncertainty. Others of us find nonspiritual ways to cope with distress and uncertainty. Mostly, though, we count on whatever qualities we can find within ourselves to help us respond to the changes that MS visits upon us.

Many of the changes we handle come as a result of what MS does *to* us. But we also must come to terms with another group of shifts—those that result from what we do *with* MS. There hasn't (to my knowledge) been any definitive study of the effects of one's attitude on the course of one's MS, although testimonial evidence abounds. People have written books or developed marketing strategies claiming that certain ways of thinking cured them of their illnesses and can cure *you* as well. I can't say what the absolute truth of such claims might be. But I do think that each of us can use shifts in attitude to affect our *feelings* about the course of the disease. I think of Kathleen Wilson, the founder of MSWorld, the online support organization for people dealing with

MS where I host a chat. Her motto is "Wellness is a state of mind." Certainly, she doesn't mean that thinking you are well will make you well absolutely (I know this because I've discussed it with her). More to the point for Ms. Wilson is that a positive attitude makes you *feel* better. Feeling better generates an energy of its own, and can carry you quite far indeed.

I don't know that a positive attitude means that you need to be uncompromisingly cheerful all the time. Nor does it necessarily mean that you should feel empowered every moment of the day. In fact, I believe that each of us determines what a "positive attitude" is for ourselves. Making those determinations and deciding to live by them, we shift attitudinal gears as we negotiate our way through the aforementioned desert.

When my MS first became symptomatic, I did not have a positive attitude à la Ms. Wilson. I had a certain amount of depression and a bit of not terribly honest holier-than-thou acceptance of my MS. I was frightened of becoming helpless and dependent on caregivers. I was terrified of losing touch with the healthy people in my life because I could no longer join them in their social, mostly physical, activities. And I did not believe medication could help me. My spiritual life, such as it was, was devoted to experiencing grief and learning to accept loss. I was practicing to be a pleasant, competently crippled woman. I thought such a practice was my best bet to prepare for the future. Anyone who wasn't doing the same thing, I deemed either to be in complete denial (most of them) or terribly fortunate (those who were in remission). I could have cruised along with that attitude forever, I suppose. It was a peaceful attitude, an accepting one. Peace and acceptance are positive qualities. For whatever reasons, though, I decided I wanted things to be different—I wanted *me* to be different. I'm sure that each of you has made similar sorts of changes as you came to terms with what MS was going to mean in *your* life.

Among the many behavioral changes I made were these: I researched the available therapies and began using the ones I felt would serve me best. I investigated mobility equipment and learned to use a variety of them (some before they were absolutely necessary, so that I would feel less helpless if they *became* absolutely necessary). I encouraged people to include me socially whenever possible, and I made sure to be a pleasant companion when I was included. If sitting and watching were all I could do, then I *chose* to sit and watch warmly and caringly. I'd found a competent counselor and I *chose* to take my anger, resentment, grief, and fear to that person rather than to share it with friends who could only be dismayed by it. Additionally, I *chose* to view my MS in terms of all the symptoms I did not have, rather than those that I did. I keep emphasizing the word "*chose*" because it did not come naturally to me to behave in these ways. I had to keep making the choices—and still have to make them. It's reassuring to find that I can still make *behavioral* choices, even though my choices are compromised in areas of *physical* ability. The choices one can make have a great influence on the experience of reality and quality of life.

So, here's the deal—I feel better. Am I *objectively* better? I neither know nor care. I'm not recommending any particular behavior as far as "positive attitude" goes. I *am* suggesting that we can *choose to pay attention* to what we are thinking or feeling about MS in our lives at any given moment. We can decide whether we want to think or feel as we do. We can decide to think or feel differently. I believe it may be the choosing *itself* that strengthens and affords some healing, no matter *what* is chosen. The positive attitude I'm talking about consists, simply, in making those choices. Happy motoring!

Acme Bowling Balls

EARLY ON A SPRING NIGHT, Twink and I were invited to join a group for a bowling party. The bowling alleys of my youth had plain wooden lanes, uncomfortable plastic seats, and large paper scoring sheets filled in by hand with arcane symbols, clumsily projected overhead when the leagues played. In contrast, the bowling alley to which we were invited that night, several miles from Cripple Creek, looked like a dance club. Dark with lots of glowing neon, the place had glittering mirrored balls overhead and the lanes were lined with flashing lights that changed color and were timed to the thumping beat of the *techno pop* pumped throughout the building. The seats were comfortably ergonomic. The scoring was computerized and displayed on monitors overhead, complete with animated graphics.

It had been years since I'd bowled, and I'd never been a very *good* bowler. In fact, it had taken me most of my teens to learn to walk swiftly to the delivery point while, at the same time, preparing to release the ball. It had taken me even longer to learn that the ball would go in the direction my thumb was pointing *at the moment of release* and not *just after release*. With weak wrists, aiming the ball had always remained difficult for me. I'd spent a number of years employed in social services. As part of my duties, I sometimes took emotionally disturbed adults and those with mental retardation on recreational bowling outings. I'd come to think of bowling as an activity for the otherwise difficult-to-occupy. It was never my first choice when seeking entertainment for myself.

On *this* night, however, I was enchanted by the atmosphere at the bowling alley. With the lights flashing and the music blaring, one could almost be inclined to *dance* to the head of the alley before delivering the ball. No longer able to dance even unencumbered by a bowling ball, I wondered what I was going to do. Someone found me a six-pound ball, the lightest one available, and I picked it up and headed toward the top of the lane. I took a stance near the end of the ball-return and held the ball as in days of old. I tried to feel for my old skip-step-slide approach but quickly realized my balance was too compromised. Instead, I walked sedately to the head of the lane, swung my arm back, delivered the ball, and watched it creep down the lane. As has been usual with me all my adult life, I took only a few pins down. But I was happy to be bowling instead of sitting on the bench. The rest of our group did, indeed, dance lightly and bowl accurately and with strength. My companions, with the exception of Twink, did not know I have MS, and I continued my slow-but-steady, low-scoring way through the first several frames. Finally someone asked me, *"Are you particularly tired this evening?"* So I explained that I have MS. What followed reminded me of the part in Menotti's opera, "Amahl and the Night Visitors," when the crippled boy throws down his crutch and takes his first unassisted steps as the Three Wise Men sing, *"He walks! He waaalks! He waaaalks!"* My friends fell back in amazement, *"She bowls! She bowls! She bowls!"* they told one another with increasing excitement. *"Isn't she amazing!"* one of them said to Twink, who beamed and acknowledged that it was so. I half-expected to see the news of my accomplishment flashed on the TV monitor overhead. I went on to bowl two games. As I did *not* when healthy, I did not bowl well on *this* occasion. But I was content with my low scores and felt no pressure to improve because, on *this* occasion, everyone, myself included, was amazed that I could bowl at *all*. *"I went bowling!"* I chirped happily all the way home.

The freedom to be poor at bowling was a new and welcome experience to me, because it was not so in my childhood. My parents were both champion league-bowlers, and the shelves in our rec-room were filled with their trophies. Taken along to bowling alleys from an early age, I was, at first, parked in the nursery with the other bowlers' little ones. As we grew through the years, we kids were free to roam, with quarters in our pockets, from the pinball arcade to the snack-bar and back, interminably it seemed, while our folks bowled. Our big treat came at the end of the evening when, the competition over, we were allowed to throw a few down the lane. Bowling doesn't require great athleticism, but it does ask strength, coordination, and a good aim of its participants. What a disappointment I was! As a child, I had poor vision, was skinny and not terribly strong, quick but uncoordinated. I wasn't a *horrible* athlete—merely a very inadequate one. With my long, thin arms, lack of coordination, poor eyesight, and stoked on sugared snacks, I excitedly and invariably bounced the ball off the alley and into the gutter. *"Aim the ball straight! Don't turn your wrist! Point your thumb at the pins! Don't lob the ball! Use the marks!"* a confusing medley of encouraging adult voices instructed from behind. My sister, stronger and sturdier than I, although three years my junior, was able to knock the pins down. As the tones of the adult chorus changed from encouraging to frustrated, I continued my failure to connect with the pins in any meaningful way.

Each week, I went home ashamed. I began to feel not terribly fond of bowling.

During my childhood, my family lived in a split-level house, one among identical hundreds, at the top of a steep hill. Across the street was a neighbor who seemed always to be peering avidly at our doings through her livingroom's picture window, which mirrored our own. My father, undoubtedly, took her interest as his due. He was a handsome man, used to women finding him fascinating and appealing. He loved being the center of admiring attention although, short of stature, he also had a small man's easily injured dignity. One evening, as spring edged into summer, and following my parents' enjoyment of after-work cocktails, my father gathered the family to see a new bowling ball that he'd brought home for the first time. Now, as you might imagine, a bowling ball is not a terribly fascinating object to view (especially in the days when they came only in basic black), particularly for two children who did not bowl. But he was very proud of his new possession, and we dutifully assembled in the living room as he lifted the ball out of its bag and held it worshipfully aloft. Mom sat in a leather butterfly chair, Sis and I sat on the floor, and we all watched as Dad took a few practice swings. Holding the ball as if to deliver, he drew his arm back and swung it forward, stopping short of letting it go. He did this two more times. The last time he did it, something went terribly wrong (depending on your idea of "wrong"). The ball left his fingers on the forward swing, flew across the room, and crashed through the picture window.

In the stunned silence that immediately followed, my mother, aware of her husband's need to be taken seriously in all circumstances, contained her response for about a split second. Then the first gurgle of amusement escaped her lips. Next, a cackle, which built to a roar. Finally, she shrieked with laughter while my sister and I watched in goggle-eyed wonder, amazed that grownups could behave this way. Still laughing, she got up from her seat and raced upstairs. My father headed out the front door, followed by my sister and me. He looked for his ball among the foundation-plantings beneath our shattered picture window but it wasn't there. He glanced toward the street and there—at her post in her own picture window—was our neighbor, her constant vigilance finally justified, smugly and silently pointing downhill. So, down the steep hill ran my father, all the way to the Rose Tree Swim Club located at the very bottom of our street. The new bowling ball had come to rest in the kiddies' wading pool. It had apparently banked off the street curb, caromed off the chain link fence at the club's entrance, and taken a dive into the pool. My sister and I had just seen several things in a few short minutes that we'd heretofore thought happened only in cartoons. We were awestruck. We now had empirical knowledge that those animated confections were based on reality and were *not* the made-up stories adults (*"don't try this at home"*) had always claimed. Our respect for our parents, particularly Father, greatly increased and my previously negative attitude toward bowling moderated somewhat.

My recent bowling experience with friends gave proof that MS has now made it blessedly impossible ever to meet my parents' inculcated expectations for me as a bowler. I feel completely purged of any lingering onus to try. But the incapacitating *shame*

I suffered over my incompetence vanished long ago, as I stood with my father beside the kiddie pool at the Rose Tree Swim Club. Through years of low-scoring games filled with gutter-balls I've been able to shrug and remind myself I am the child of a man who can handle a bowling ball with the finesse of Wiley Coyote.

The Abyss

THOSE OF US WITH MS are often advised to keep our spirits up. And, as I've written, many who have the disease attribute their relative well-being to the adoption of a positive attitude. When I was first diagnosed, I entered immediately into a state of denial and, thus, seemed to be "taking it well." This was not a positive attitude, although it probably protected me from developing a negative one. But once denial was no longer possible, and I realized I had an incurable, progressive disease, it was necessary that I find my way through my own darkness and my experience of MS into that positive place. I don't particularly adhere to a strict order for the stages of response to personal disaster, but I did need to grieve and to be angry. I needed to deny and to try to weasel my way out of the situation—all this before I could even *begin* groping toward peace, contentment, acceptance and, finally, joy.

For me, weaseling and denial went hand in hand. When first diagnosed, I took the news calmly. I'd never paid disabled people much attention, and I knew nothing about MS. I was an active woman and, although I'd played a good game of recreational volleyball up until then, I left the hospital where the diagnosis took place and joined a highly competitive, touring, power volleyball team. I was very gung-ho, played through any injuries, and ran the legs off my teammates like some distressing combination of Gidget and G.I. Joe. In between games, I was fatigued, walked with a cane, and generally acted out of deep reserves of neediness. Among my main concerns, as if disease could be a fashion accessory, was whether becoming disabled would make me *more*, or *less*, socially attractive. I reflected upon sick or injured heroines in operas and storybooks—beautiful women stoically suffering their fates, each with a despairing but care-taking true love at her side. At that time in my life, I was fairly extreme and thought I had either to be in excellent health, brimming with vitality and demonstrating it constantly or else the best damned cripple the world had ever seen. My initial symptoms disappeared relatively quickly and I "forgot" I had MS for many years.

Remember those cartoons in which a character runs off a cliff and keeps going, legs churning in mid-air over the chasm? When he notices he's no longer on solid ground he plummets. I was like that character for a long time, until my symptoms reasserted themselves. I searched through many possible explanations for what I was experiencing. I tried to correct for my deficits with diet, different clothing, and more exercise. I investigated carpal-tunnel syndrome, vitamin B deficiency, and allergies. I didn't consider MS as the cause of my difficulties. I disowned the parts of me that were failing. It wasn't *my* leg that was dragging. It was *that darned leg*! *Those* numb fingers were not *mine*. Things hit home for me one day out cross-country skiing with friends. In the past, I'd enjoyed gliding over the ground on my skis, but on this day I realized I couldn't feel the ground well enough to make the necessary adjustments that allow skiing to be such a pleasure. I had to head for the lodge while my friends stayed on the trail. I was angry with my body, angry with my friends for being able to continue on, and scared. Thus, began my plummet into the abyss.

Although each of us has his own, all abysses seem to have certain features in common. All seem to be made up, in part, of unresolved longings and conflicts from our pasts. All seem to be repositories for aspects of our character that we wish to disown. The time I spent in my own darkness has proved itself very valuable to me.

Once I knew myself to be falling, it became important to prepare for a landing. I began to educate myself, as well as those who loved me, about MS. I also found a neurologist with whom I could work and a psychotherapist. Of the two, the psychotherapist proved the more important. It has been observed that the profoundly mentally ill are often able to survive a disaster by pulling themselves together, only to collapse back into their sickness once the disaster has passed. Although I was nowhere near to being that disturbed, like most people, I had been trudging along with my negative baggage intact, dumping it here and there as conflicts presented themselves. MS was my wake-up call. I understood that my successful survival as a disabled person might hinge on a deeper awareness of motivations—both my own and those of people caring for me, should such care become necessary. Faced with the possibility of becoming *truly* needy, I could no longer afford *not* to explore and resolve the dysfunctional emotional needs I'd heretofore romanticized.

I fell through my abyss for several years. I despaired of myself and of my willingness to live with increasing disability. Formerly a champion of my own neediness, I now expressed worry over becoming a burden to others. I had thoughts of suicide, especially should I become incapacitated and confined to a wheelchair. When I look back at that time from my *current* perspective, I'm struck by how self-centered my concerns were. I was deeply ashamed of myself for becoming, as I saw it, less-than-acceptable physically. And, far from *really* objecting to others having to look after me, I was scared of being a person who needed looking after. What a blow to my self-esteem that would be! And *what if there was no one who wanted to do it?*

Then there were the losses. No longer able to participate in sports as I had, no longer having the dexterity to play a musical instrument well, I had to grieve. Much of my sense of self, and some of my livelihood, had come from those two activities. I haunted my abyss, feeling useless and as if *nothing* mattered. Again, this was a selfish attitude insofar as my personal situation still represented the entire world to me. I have a friend with terminal cancer who has told me that she sees more outside herself now than when she had no notion of dying. She stands and stares at trees, even in winter, and sees them as *trees,* with no relation or comparison to her own journey toward death. But I could do no such thing.

As I worked on these issues in therapy, I gradually found myself better able to face and handle the challenges of MS. I became more confident and less conflicted as I handled some of those challenges successfully or, at least, more gracefully than I otherwise would have. I became less needy within and more accepting of whatever my needs might actually be in the present. I began to find things I could do—and enjoyed doing—that were different from things I'd done and enjoyed before MS. Some of these activities I would never have tried in the past because, then, I wasn't a person who *enjoyed* such activities. But now I had *no idea* who I was. With no preconceptions, I was free to allow a new self to come into being.

When I began to experience disability due to MS, I was advised by others with the disease to let go of things that didn't matter, to prioritize in order to conserve energy. They were speaking of things such as household tasks and unwanted social obligations. But the main thing that I discovered didn't matter was *me*. I don't mean this in a negative, sad way. I mean that who-I-thought-I-had-to-be was only an idea in my mind and not a reality engraved in stone. And with the blessed experience of *that* realization, I was able to begin my climb out of the abyss.

There are so *many* ways to climb back to solid ground. I used psychotherapy and a spiritual program of recovery, among other methods, but there are other spiritual paths both organized and individual, there are relationships with people and activities of all kinds, there are writers whose words enlighten and motivate, and there are simply those chance occurrences that are called by the words *kismet, grace, serendipity, fate*—experiences that open us in a profound way, freeing us from the prison of our perceptions. That prison itself sets each of us up for the eventual fall into the abyss, and it seems that the abysmal experience is necessary before each of us can rise again to embrace life with clarity. But many of us do.

It's a cold, rainy spring day as I write this here at Cripple Creek. The gray of the sky and the drab browns left from the recent winter accentuate the intense green of tiny nascent leaves on the bushes outside my window. All of us with MS have lives well worth living. I believe there is a winter within each of us that can, in time, give way to spring.

The Red Pony

ACROSS THE ROAD from Cripple Creek is a farm owned by a man who rescues livestock from laboratories. He mainly takes in sheep and goats, which he then raises for their wool. On any day, I can see him zooming around on his all-terrain vehicle (ATV) as he tends to his charges. He's especially busy in spring, when the sheep and goats have their babies. I've always enjoyed watching the young ones cavort in the barnyard, and I've accepted the annoying sound of his ATV because I know he's using it to save him steps in his farm work.

One day about six years ago, I stood leaning on my cane observing the lambs and kids. I was very tired from having walked a quarter-mile to do some repair work near where our properties abut. With my weak and spastic legs, walking this far had become very difficult and, as my neighbor sped past, I wondered whether a machine such as his might be a good idea for me. But I discarded the idea quickly. I didn't want the noise or the smell of a gas-powered ATV disturbing the peace of Cripple Creek.

Back home, I considered electric scooters. But many of them have only three wheels and, even with four, most of them are made for (as the catalogs say) "smoothly groomed" surfaces. There are almost no smoothly groomed surfaces on this farm-become-nature-sanctuary, and the few that there are do not take me where I wish or need to go. There were two interesting scooters, though, made for hunters and fishermen. I thought perhaps one of them would do and called a local company that sells mobility equipment to explain my needs to them. Because they *are* a local company, they understand farms. The scooters in which I was interested have knobby tires for rough surfaces, I was told, but lack the power for hills and rocky terrain. Instead, they suggested a scooter with knobby tires that also had a four-wheel-drive. The next day they brought one over for a test-ride. It was big, and a shiny, candy-apple red. It went up steep hills, drove easily over stones and uncut grass, handled six-inch drop-offs, and could even be used in a few inches of snow.

When I was very young, like many other little girls, I wanted a pony. I read about ponies, collected horse figurines, and galloped around the yard hitting my thigh with a twig while leaping over upturned patio furniture. I snorted, tossed my head, whickered, and stamped my sneakered foot. Fantasy-ponies took up most of my imagination, but what I wanted, of course, was a *real* one. I never got one, though. Instead, as my parents one day gaily informed me, I was to have a *little sister*! "*Big deal*," I reflected, sourly. When she arrived I called her "The Pony Who Couldn't Do *Anything*" (of which name, to this day, no-one in my family, least of all my sister, understands the meaning).

By middle-age, I assumed I'd outgrown my pony-lust. But one trip on the bright red scooter brought it all back. I was encouraged by friends with MS to give my scooter a name. Remembering the title of a Steinbeck horse-story from my childhood (without, thankfully, remembering the content), I dubbed my scooter the *Red Pony*.

I built Red Pony a stall in the barn. Intended for outdoor use, it's too big to be in the house, although just like a real pony, it needs shelter from precipitation and the cold winters. I put a shelf in the stall to hold the battery-charger, electricity being this "pony's" grain. A plastic air-conditioner cover did admirably for a rain-fly against moisture blowing in from outside and, for really cold nights in the barn, I used an electric blanket under the plastic cover to keep the batteries warm. Like the child Jody in Steinbeck's novella did with his Gabilan, I took good care of my own Red Pony. I kept it well-charged, the deck brushed free of debris, the chrome shined, and the body sparkling clean.

With the cloth seat covered against the wet, and the handlebars equally protected by a rain bonnet, Red Pony and I set out to explore parts of Cripple Creek to which I hadn't been in years. What a sense of freedom I had! What joy it was to ride along, the breeze in my face, the quiet hum of electric motors in my ears. I visited places I'd used to walk to regularly to enjoy the wildflowers. I was glad to find the flowers were still there. I found the homes of animals I used to keep an eye on—squirrels, groundhogs, and such. Many were still in use. In other places, changes had occurred: a stream had altered its course slightly, a tree had come down. In those areas, I had to reacquaint myself, learning what lived there now and what had moved on. Birds, which ordinarily flee at the approach of a human, didn't recognize my form on Red Pony and, with my binoculars along, I was able to add several new ones to the list I keep.

The only problem involved the multiflora rose bushes that abound on Cripple Creek. They are gorgeous in bloom, provide food for animals in fall and winter, and shed thorns all year long. My poor "pony" kept getting thorns in its little pneumatic "hooves." Then I'd have to leave it in the pasture, the woods, or wherever we happened to be, and walk home to call the mobility service to come and "vet" it. This was not a very secure feeling and, the third time it occurred, I asked for foam inserts for the tires. The ride became a little harder on the tail-bone, but I was assured of being able to return home.

When people came to visit, I was now able to accompany them on long "walks" about the place instead of sending them out and waiting at home myself. On the Red Pony, I was able to do a larger variety of chores on my own instead of having to ask someone else to do them. I trained my two small terriers to ride on the deck so that they could go along with me. I was even able to carry loads on the deck of the Red Pony that an able-bodied person could not have carried. This made me useful to others on Cripple Creek in a way I'd not experienced for some time. It was a good feeling and it continued for several years.

It would be a good feeling still, except that I began enjoying something of a remission in my MS. I found I could walk to places to which I used to have to ride. For a while, I continued to keep the "pony" well-groomed and charged in case I needed it. But my legs grew stronger. This fall, as in past years, I covered the Red Pony and turned on the electric blanket so that the batteries would work as the weather cooled. By mid-winter, I had not used it for months, so I disconnected the batteries and brought them inside for the winter. These days, the Red Pony stands abandoned in the stall. The plastic covers are put away, for there are no batteries to protect. I don't spend time brushing the carpeted deck, shining the chrome, or polishing its fender-flanks anymore.

But spring is here. There will be wildflowers to visit and migrating birds to observe. And, as is often the case with my MS, I find myself experiencing a slight flare-up—not enough to alarm me, but enough to, perhaps, warrant the resurrection of the Red Pony. In the next week or so, as the weather warms, I plan to reinstall the batteries, shake out and vacuum the deck's carpeting, replace the plastic seat and faring covers, and generally spruce things up. I may even invite the mobility equipment folks out to give it the once-over. And then, if everything checks out, I'll be back in the saddle again. Off we'll go, the Red Pony and I, and you may imagine us heading off into a warm, vernal sunset somewhere on Cripple Creek.